Rapid weight loss hypnosis

&

Gastric band hypnosis

eat healthy stop sugar cravings exploits psychology meditation & mindful to prevent disease through self esteem and self control

Charlotte brown

TABLE OF CONTENTS

Gastric band
hypnosis

INTRODUCTION

Overweight people are continually looking for ways that support them on their weight loss journey. Still, many are hesitant to go for traditional gastric band procedures to establish a healthier relationship with food. Hypnosis for weight loss thus provides a feasible option that's healthy and very inexpensive.

Weight loss hypnotherapy has become more common and readily accessible over the past few years. People recognize the many distinct, beneficial effects of hypnotherapy and, as a result, are becoming less skeptical of these styles of treatments.

Hypnosis is a state of mind that simply occurs; it's the same state of deep relaxation you experience when you're about to fall asleep at night. It can also happen when you dream, listen to music or watch an excellent movie: you can become oblivious of what is going on around you when you concentrate intensely on something unique, or how much time has elapsed.

Gastric band hypnotherapy is the therapeutic use of hypnosis, which is typically done in a psychiatric setting to help people make meaningful changes which progress in specific areas of their life. A hypnotherapist uses worded ideas to help you solve particular challenges, such as modifying and breaking an unhelpful habit, like smoking, for example, or even chewing your nails. Hypnotherapy can also be used to help you let go of negative views, to build a more optimistic self-image, increase your self-esteem, and boost your self-confidence. The people who are taking part in the programme must want to make these changes and trust in their abilities to do it too, for the hypnotherapy to be as successful as possible.

But how does this weight loss hypnosis Hypnotherapy work in

the field of weight loss? Research findings also support the argument that using hypnotherapy/hypnosis in weight loss can be highly successful and help develop a healthier relationship with your food; in reality, it is comparable to the gastric band in terms of success. You should read the abstracts Efficacy of hypnosis as an adjunct to behavioral weight management and also a Regulated trial of hypnotherapy for weight loss in patients with obstructive sleep apnoea.

Chapter 1: UNDERSTANDING HYPNOSIS

What about hypnosis?

Hypnosis is a mental condition that is trance-like, in which people undergo heightened concentration, focus, and suggestibility. While hypnosis is often characterized as a state of sleep, it is better represented as a state of intense attention, increased suggestibility, and vivid fantasies. People sometimes seem sleepy and zoned out in a hypnotic state, but they are in a hyper-awareness state.

Hypnosis is a very real technique used as a therapeutic method, but there are many myths and misconceptions. It has been shown that hypnosis has medical and psychological effects, most importantly in reducing pain and anxiety. It has also been proposed that the symptoms of dementia may be decreased by hypnosis.

Hypnosis Forms

There are a few different forms of administering hypnosis:

- Directed hypnosis: This type of hypnosis involves using instruments to induce a hypnotic state, such as recorded instructions and music. Web sites and mobile apps mostly use this method of hypnosis.
- Hypnotherapy: Hypnotherapy is hypnosis in psychotherapy and is utilized to treat depression, anxiety, post-traumatic stress disorder (PTSD), and eating disorders by licensed clinicians and psychologists.
- Self-hypnosis: Self-hypnosis is a process that occurs when a hypnotic state is self-induced by an individual. It is also used as a self-help tool for pain relief or stress management.

Utilizations

Why should a person decide to try hypnosis? In certain cases, to help cope with chronic pain or relieve pain and anxiety caused by medical procedures such as surgery or childbirth, people may seek hypnosis.

The following are only a few of the hypnosis applications that have been seen through research: 3

- Alleviation of irritable bowel syndrome (IBS) related symptoms
  - Pain management during dental procedures
- Elimination or elimination, including warts and psoriasis, of skin conditions
- Control of such ADHD symptoms
- Treatment of problems with chronic pain such as rheumatoid arthritis
- Treatment and pain relief during childbirth 4
- Reduction in signs of dementia
- Reduction of nausea and vomiting of patients with cancer who undergo chemotherapy

Hypnosis has also been used to assist individuals with improvements in behavior, such as stopping smoking, losing weight, or avoiding bed-wetting.

Hypnosis Effect

What's the effect of hypnosis? The hypnosis experience can differ significantly from one person to another.

During the hypnotic state, some hypnotized people report experiencing a sense of isolation or intense relaxation, while others also believe like their acts appear to occur outside of their conscious will. Although under hypnosis, other people can remain fully conscious and able to carry out conversations.

Researcher Ernest Hilgard's tests revealed how hypnosis could be used to significantly change perceptions.5 The participant's arm was then put in ice water after instructing a hypnotized person not to experience discomfort in their arm. While non-hypnotized individuals had to withdraw their arm from the water after a few seconds because of the discomfort, without experiencing pain, the hypnotized individuals were able to keep their arms in the freezing water for many minutes.

What feels like hypnosis?

Tips

While many individuals assume they can not be hypnotized, research has shown that a significant number of individuals are more hypnotized than they realize. It is proposed by studies that:

About 10% and 15% of individuals are very sensitive to hypnosis.

Around 10% of adults are known to be difficult or impossible to hypnotize.

Kids appear to be more sensitive to hypnosis.

Hypnosis is often more sensitive to individuals who can be readily consumed in fantasies.

It's important to note approaching the process with an open mind if you're interested in being hypnotized. People who positively perceive hypnosis appear to have a stronger response.

It is important to look for a doctor who has qualifications and experience in hypnosis as a therapeutic device if you are interested in seeking hypnotherapy.

It might be beneficial to search for a mental health professional that has been trained by the American Society of Clinical Hypnosis, but several sites offer hypnosis training and certification. Their program is open to master's degree health practitioners and includes 40 hours of licensed workshop training, 20 hours of individual training, and two years of clinical hypnosis practice.

Potential Pitfalls

It is normal to have misunderstandings about the topic of hypnosis.

Although in extremely rare cases, amnesia may occur, people usually remember all that happened when they were hypnotized. Hypnosis may, however, have a major impact on memory. Posthypnotic amnesia may cause a person to forget certain things that happened before or during hypnosis. This impact is, however, usually restricted and temporary.

Although hypnosis may be used to improve memory, the effects of mass media have been greatly exaggerated. Research has shown that hypnosis does not contribute to substantial change or consistency in memory, and hypnosis can lead to false or distorted memories.

Hypnosis does require voluntary intervention on the part of the patient, despite reports regarding people being hypnotized without their consent. However, people differ in terms of how hypnotizable and suggestible they are when they are under hypnosis. Research shows that strongly suggestible individuals when under hypnosis, are more likely to feel a decreased sense of agency.

Although people often believe that without the power of their will, their actions under hypnosis tend to occur, a hypnotist can not make you do actions against your wishes.

Although it is possible to use hypnosis to boost results, it does not make people stronger or more athletic than their current physical abilities.

The Hypnosis History

The use of hypnotic-like trance states goes back thousands of years, but from a physician called Franz Mesmer, hypnosis started to emerge during the late 18th century. Thanks to Mesmer's spiritual beliefs, the activity got off to a poor start, but attention gradually moved to a more scientific approach.

In the late 19th-century, hypnotism became more relevant in psychology and was used by Jean-Martin Charcot to treat women suffering what was then known as hysteria. This work inspired Sigmund Freud and the development of psychoanalysis.

More recently, to clarify precisely how hypnosis operates, there have been a variety of different hypotheses. Hilgard's neo-dissociation theory of hypnosis is one of the best-known theories. 10

People in a hypnotic state undergo a split consciousness in which there are two separate sources of mental activity, according to Hilgard. Although one stream of consciousness responds to the suggestions of the hypnotist, another dissociated stream processes knowledge outside of the conscious awareness of the hypnotized person.

Losing weight can be a daunting task not made any easier by the contradictory advice out there in the world, and sometimes risky. With TV shows, ads, and social media feed full of food photos, we are constantly bombarded, and the existence of these can make the desire to shift away from safe or intuitive eating very powerful.

Then there are pills for weight loss and other plans for commercial weight control that focus on minimizing what you consume instead of contemplating how you consume or what you think about the food you put into your body. It is no wonder that certain harmful mindsets have formed around what we put in our bodies.

Weight loss hypnosis can be a successful way to question these mental behaviors and moments of temptation, encouraging you to live a healthy life.

The purpose of weight loss hypnotherapy is to make you feel good about your body, shift unhealthy eating thoughts, and help you responsibly lose weight without affecting your emotional well-being. A hypnotherapist can help you build a healthier relationship with food and exercise, which is essential to safe weight loss and long-term weight control by engaging the unconscious mind with effective suggestion techniques.

Is it important for me to lose weight?

Many people, whether they are overweight or not, insist that they need to lose weight. But the fact is, very few individuals, regardless of whether they need to lose weight, are content with the shape and size of their bodies.

More specifics on weight loss can be found at Nutritionist Resource.

Trust in the body

Although individuals must lose weight if they are overweight for health reasons, it's not good to feel ashamed of the need or urge to lose weight. Since body shape and size are so connected to the western definition of beauty, people are constantly searching for 'fast fixes' to cut corners.

Any of the ways people attempt to lose weight are weight loss supplements, fad diets, and grueling workout regimes. What do you need to ask yourself is-am I happy to do this? For the rest of my life, can I continue doing this?

This is where weight loss hypnotherapy can improve. You need to first change your mind to change your body. Why am I dissatisfied with my body, and why can't I lose weight? You must ask yourself.

Visit our fact sheet to read more about how low self-confidence can be improved by hypnotherapy.

How does weight loss hypnosis work?

Hypnotherapy for weight loss is becoming more common, and it is good for maintaining a healthy weight in the long term for people all over the world.

Over time, you will learn how to substitute your negative habits and to eat behaviors with healthy ones recommended by your hypnotherapist-and a series of weight loss hypnotherapy sessions.

What occurs during weight loss hypnosis?

You will be directed into a state of deep relaxation by your hypnotherapist.

Your hypnotherapist will be able to reach your unconscious mind until your body and mind are completely relaxed (the part of us that operates all the time but that we are not aware of, i.e., instincts and survival mechanisms).

It is possible to use relaxing, carefully worded scripts to discuss why a client overeats and proposes new ways of thinking through visualizations. Without any input from your hypnotherapist, you can ignore any suggestions you don't feel comfortable with. For some of the strategies and visualizations they can use, see below.

Hypnotherapy for techniques to lose weight

While each scenario is different and everyone has their reasons for wanting to lose weight, some suggestions that you might find include:

- Imagining the body you want or the fitness/health standard you want to attain.
- Imagining how your new look and wellbeing would make you feel.
- Imagining yourself comfortably hitting that target.
- See how far from today you would have changed.
- Imagine how energized and safe you would feel.

Realizing that the more you workout, the more you want to workout, and the harder it will become to do so.

These strategies are meant to motivate you so that you can take charge of your decisions. However, if you're worried that your relationship with certain food types is becoming unhealthy, hypnotherapy for food addiction could help you break these cycles of negative thinking.

You can learn to love the taste of healthy food by weight loss hypnosis, and avoid wanting sugary, fatty foods. You should also learn and not see it as a source of distress to love your body. Hypnosis for weight loss will help you follow a healthy lifestyle and a happier attitude by confronting those deep emotions that form the pillars of your eating habits.

Your Weight Loss Possible Blocks

For a variety of reasons, plenty of individuals attempt and struggle to lose weight. These causes are mostly unconscious, often referred to as 'secondary benefits,' making it impossible for us to resolve them.

It is worth looking at the confidence that has held the weight in place for so long when someone loses weight. We always hold beliefs at two levels; we think positive thoughts about ourselves, our worth, and what we deserve as human beings at the conscious level; but our behaviors unconsciously give away our emotional beliefs.

-- Amreeta Chapman / Aujayeb, a clinical hypnotherapist, discusses the issues that people can face while trying to lose weight.

The fact is, by not making changes, we can sometimes gain security-we feel comfortable remaining just as we are. So, we may want to lose weight consciously, but something in the subconscious is keeping us from making it a reality. Weight loss hypnotherapy seeks to uncover these causes, helping consumers to eventually push through obstacles that could have stopped them from losing weight for several years.

You eat comfort from food

We learn to equate feeding with the warmth of our mothers

when we are infants. Some experts believe that this connection never really leaves us, so we can return to those early days of total dependence when life gets stressful. This is where it can become an issue for emotional eating.

If you have ever found yourself after a long day reaching for a chocolate bar, or ordering a takeaway when you feel lonely and sad, then you could be a comfort eater. You would find it harder to lose weight as a comfort eater because you have let food become your coping mechanism, and, without it, you do not know how to cope with your emotions.

Hypnotherapy will help fix this, allowing you to understand how negative feelings are handled in a way that does not contribute to eating comfort.

The biggest change is that I have been much less bothered to eat. I love it, but when my body is hungry, I have learned to feed, not only because my mind needs anything to soothe my feelings.

— Julia shares how emotional eating was overcome by hypnotherapy.

You're eating mindlessly,

You have to be frank about how much you eat and exercise to lose weight. It's easy to forget about the occasional snack here and there, even though you keep a food diary or use a food-tracking app. Maybe you choose ingredients when you're making dinner? Do you catch something on your ride to work, or do you tuck your afternoon tea into a biscuit?

These 'on the go' foods are always those that catch us out. However, they add up. Even if you diligently stick to salad for dinner, it won't do you any favors to conveniently forget all the things you eat in between. This sort of mindless eating is something weight loss hypnotherapy can help you to resolve.

If you struggle with conscious feeding, gastric band

hypnotherapy might help you. The intention is to make you feel fuller for longer, which may help stop excessive day-long grazing.

You're banning food

Like a mystery package, you're told not to open; it can make them all the more desirable by removing those foods from your diet. If you find yourself limiting the foods you consume, when your willpower takes a dip, you're more likely to want to binge.

Learning to eat attentively is the secret to sustainable and effective weight loss. You'll be able to enjoy your favorite foods in moderation and stop piling on weight if you can eat carefully, savoring every bite.

A vital aspect of weight loss hypnosis is encouraging consumers to eat deliberately-setting aside emotional factors and cultivating a stable relationship with food that encourages a long-term, healthy weight.

You're not exercising sufficiently

When it comes to weight loss, exercise is just as important as diet. Mental blocks can often stop us wanting to exercise, including:

- Feeling an absence of resources
- Feeling too self-conscious to publicly exercise
- Persuading yourself that you're going to 'go tomorrow' (every day)

Hypnotherapy for weight loss will help you break down the mental blocks that stop you from making the most of your body. In general, keeping your body working and your heart pumping can help you feel better about yourself more often than not, contributing to healthy habits and long-term satisfaction.

Will weight loss hypnosis work out for me?

In hypnotherapy sessions, one of the most frequently asked questions is-can weight loss hypnotherapy function for me? The response to that is, before you try it yourself, it's hard to tell. While it definitely won't work the same way for everybody, when it comes to diet and exercise, the process of talking about creating healthy habits and getting rid of poor habits can help to build a new level of knowledge.

Hypnotherapy is supportive treatment, an vital point to remember, and can also be used with a balanced eating plan and exercise routine. You can find it helpful to talk to your doctor or nutrition professional if you want advice about eating healthy and exercising. With all these aspects, it is always a joint effort that contributes to results.

Chapter 2: THE FOUNDATIONS OF WEIGHT LOSS

Achieving quick and efficient fat loss involves the combined effects of many different approaches. Follow these 12 main factors for sustained and consistent fat loss performance.

Achieving quick and successful fat loss involves the combined effects of many different methods, which, when used correctly too, directly and indirectly, target excess weight, can allow one to sustain their fat loss efforts to keep the pounds off. Fast fire methods such as the "lose 10 pounds in ten days" style techniques we see too frequently across our television sets rarely work. If they do are not effective as they are simply quick solutions designed to quickly drop the fat through drastic dietary and exercise methods, which can cause harm if practiced longer than necessary.

By attempting fat loss by depriving yourself of certain nutrients or working a specific part of your body / focusing on only one training strategy, you may be risking your health in many ways. For example, a broad spectrum of nutrients is required to address the many functions our body has and a balanced training program. Combining resistance training (which focuses on working all of our muscles) and cardiovascular work is both workable over the long term and efficient for establishing a healthy, optimally functioning, and good looking body. Those that have experienced body transformation success usually have made their health and wellness a priority, one that, through the benefits reaped and ease with which it can be sustained, has easily become a lifestyle.

And therein lies the secret to long term body transformation success: prepare efficiently and weave your training goals into your day to day life. Twelve main factors have proven many to provide successful, attainable, and sustainable foundations for continued fat loss success. Use them, and you, too, will experience great health and enviable physical growth for many years to come.

FOUNDATION 1 GOALS SET

Very little can be done without a strong plan in place, regardless of what health and fitness goals one wishes to accomplish. So set aside some time to assess where you are now before setting foot inside the gym and preparing the first of your power meals as you embark on your body transformation, and contrast this with where you would like to be in, say, a year from now. Be precise with time frames and have a specified image of what you want to look like and how you want to feel at the end of your transformation. Be mindful, though, that you will need to have more goals in place after you have reached your health and fitness goals to sustain or improve on what you have already accomplished.

Document your goals and have them readily available-to verify your results; you may need to revisit them. These targets would need to be practical and achievable: developing muscles to compete with Mr. Olympia, complete with three percent levels of body fat, would probably not happen, ever, at least in this lifetime. Assess the sort of body you have and plan your objectives accordingly. Be comfortable with steady weight loss if you are severely overweight and do not get frustrated if you do not seem to lose fat fast enough.

If you follow the instructions given below, you will get the results you want. With them in mind, plan your objectives and do not stop until you have achieved your perfect physique.

FOUNDATION 2 WITH WEIGHTS

This seems quite obvious, but it's surprising how many people will concentrate primarily on aerobic activities while relegating weights to additional status when trying to lose weight. To lose body fat, cardiovascular training methods should never be used at the expense of resistance training. It is smart to build as much of it as possible to stimulate metabolic activity as frequently as possible, given the mere presence of muscle tissue significantly increases the metabolic rate, including while we are resting. We can continue the fat burning process long after our workouts by encouraging our metabolic rate-how fast. Our bodies burn energy-to work faster while we are at rest (a complete state of inactivity where only our vital organs require the release of energy).

"Weight training will lead to enhanced muscle tissue that will increase metabolism and fat loss in turn."

Through the results of many success stories of transformation, it has been shown that anaerobic training-one form is weight training-is far superior to aerobic training for increasing our basal metabolic rate (or the rate at which we burn energy when fully rested). While aerobic training will target fat while it is used, during and after its use, weight training will increase the metabolic rate and build muscle to increase our metabolic rate further. Being a metabolically active tissue, muscle requires more energy to retain than fat, useless in excess.

DO CARDIO, FOUNDATION 3

Although weight training is crucial for improving one's metabolic rate, the cardiovascular activity will also further assist fat loss efforts when used in conjunction with weights. It appears that the major issue with cardio is that it is often overused. Those desperate for fat loss will readily associate weight loss with aerobic training. If you look at the physiques of those who train aerobically exclusively, although they are usually slim, with the very little tone, they have a soft appearance.

Compare these 'athletes' with bodybuilders. You will usually see a significant difference in physical appearance: the bodybuilder will usually have lower levels of body fat and, almost always, better growth of muscles. The reason for such a difference is that with weight training, which will be prioritized ahead of aerobic activity, the bodybuilder will balance his cardio work. It is essential to include cardio at levels that target body fat without interfering with recovery from weight training workouts and muscle growth for body transformation.

A good start is three 45-minute moderate-intensity output (about 70 percent of maximum heart rate) cardio sessions per week, first on an empty stomach in the morning. To determine whether this level is appropriate for your individual needs, be sure to monitor your progress-you may need to increase or decrease this amount accordingly. You will be on the right track as long as your body fat levels drop and your body looks tighter without apparent muscle loss.

FOUNDATION 4 MAINTAIN A WELL BALANCED DIET

Steady, consistent loss of fat probably results in more than any other variable from sensible eating. As mentioned, we need to build muscle and train with weights to boost this and, directly, the metabolic process to increase one's metabolic rate to promote an around-the-clock fat-burning effect. However, we need enough high-quality nutrients interspersed throughout the day to reach the energy levels needed to maintain sufficient training intensity and to recover from our intensive workouts and grow. It is necessary to consume proteins, carbohydrates, and fats along with a wide range of vitamins and minerals and to plan a good balance for each one.

It is important to ensure that we do not consume too many of the wrong kinds of nutrients to lose body fat. When the real problem lies with the calories we consume, people often become caught up in restricting overall calories. The longing for carbohydrates that many people have is one of the major obstacles to maintaining low levels of body fat. Due to the positive effect on specific brain chemicals such as serotonin and dopamine, a nutrient that is comforting is necessary for energy production and easily stored as body fat if over-consumed. It is often difficult to strike the right balance between eating enough carbohydrates to fuel our workouts and to support day-to-day life while discouraging its conversion into body fat.

We cause insulin to be released whenever we eat too many carbohydrates-especially those that cause a rapid energy output, such as the simple variety that includes cakes, sweets, and some fruits. Which, in turn, transforms these carbohydrates into glycogen to be stored for future use. If we already have adequate glycogen stores, the problem is that any surplus will be transformed into body fat and stored as such. And this is one reason why bodybuilders, and those who want to succeed in transforming their body, often include nearly as much protein as carbohydrates in their diet.

Protein is important for the success of fat loss as a nutrient that requires more energy to process and which is instrumental in building the muscle mass needed to increase the metabolic rate. Therefore, a good diet could include about 40 percent protein calories, 45 percent carbohydrates, with the remainder coming from essential fats such as particular oils, avocado, and nuts (including olive and Omega three fish oils). Eat around six meals per day consisting of the above nutritional profile and avoid carbohydrates after 6.00 pm to further accentuate the success of fat loss.

FOUNDATION 5 HYDRATED STAY

Staying hydrated through adequate water consumption (about 15 glasses per day for the exercise enthusiast) is a great way to encourage the fat burning process and be essential for overall physical performance and health. Fat burning can only really be achieved at a fundamental level when the body is running optimally. If any of our metabolic processes are not working to their fullest, the body will place its resources to compensate for such a problem, leaving other processes to function less effectively, such as fat burning by drinking enough water, by supporting all of our body's biological functions.

For instance, muscle consists of around 75 percent water. It is not likely to exert positive metabolic effects to burn fat without enough water to support the proper functioning of this tissue muscle. Also, when aiming to transform their physiques, another problem individuals tend to have is water retention. Although not related to fat storage, water retention often results from insufficient hydration; the more water we drink, the more effectively our kidneys work, and the faster any subcutaneous water can be removed from under our skin. Thus, we can help eliminate water retention by drinking sufficiently clean, fresh water while creating the conditions necessary for continuous fat loss.

FOUNDATION 6 MAKE A LIFESTYLE FOR HEALTH AND FITNESS

Health and fitness must become a firmly entrenched part of one's lifestyle to truly experience long-term weight loss success. If you can not incorporate into your daily schedule the fundamental principles such as those outlined in this article-needed to achieve ongoing results, all the planning and goal setting in the world, along with perfectly developed training and nutritional programs, will account for very little. Waking up in the morning to finish your cardio, for instance, should ultimately come as naturally as eating your breakfast and brushing your teeth.

Do not view your goals for transformation as something that should be considered specifically outside the normal course of your daily life. It is best to structure your goals into a lifestyle that is both sustainable over the long term, and that will ultimately define who you are as an individual to make it work long-term. In essence, an inextricable component of who you are will become your health and fitness program.

FOUNDATION 7 MEASURE YOUR PROGRESS AND TAKE NOTES

Take time to weigh yourself regularly, measure your levels of body fat, and evaluate any changes in muscle growth, if appropriate and relevant. Doing so will provide you with significant information to re-evaluate your current programs and plan for even greater success. While the mirror is often considered the best friend of a bodybuilder, as this will indicate the degree of progress achieved, more objective measures such as those mentioned above will provide concrete information to gauge the true effectiveness of a program.

For instance, if your body fat levels are only marginally lower than they were four months earlier, then it's time to change one or more of the variables in your program: you may need to increase your cardio, weights, or both. Perhaps your lack of achievement might be nutritionally related. And this is why it is critical for the success of body transformation to maintain training and nutrition journals: they allow you to evaluate exactly what you have done, where you may have slacked off, and the kind of responses you experienced from a particular workout. Be sure to note any progress-however large or small in your journals and record all workouts and meals extensively.

Eventually, you may not need to use a training journal, but it remains an effective way to learn what works for you and what does not while you adjust to your new lifestyle.

FOUNDATION 8 BE CONSISTENT

Consistency is closely associated with the value of making health and fitness a lifestyle. As a rule, never missing a scheduled workout or meal is crucial. It is prudent to remain on track as long as you have arranged your meals and training in compliance with your specific requirements and in such a way as to achieve the best possible results. Although professional athletes are effectively using instinctive training strategies to promote more performance, and may even work for you sometime in the future, it is best to do what you regularly have during these early stages. During your initial goal setting, it will work best for you.

The number one reason people struggle to meet their fitness

goals is the lack of discipline they are often seen to demonstrate. Imposing high intensity during one session only to take a mental and physical break from going all-out during the next exercise would typically only result in half-hearted outcomes. These average exercises will be reflected in the results you see, combined throughout a six to 12-week program. Typically, they would then blame their software when, in fact, it is more a case of not implementing what was supposed to function properly from the outset.

Instead of modifying the program based on the mistaken presumption that there are flaws with its nature. If you fail to meet the training objectives, try to decide if you have been consistent with implementing your training and diet requirements and the commitment you have contributed to both.

FOUNDATION 9 BE CONFIDENT

Lacking confidence in your ability to lose weight would negate any attempts at fat loss. It's time to work on creating the body of your dreams after a comprehensive target setting and preparation. But how many individuals decide to slip back into old habits after suffering a loss, a phase that most eventually results in leaving one's program? Losing weight can be challenging, though possible, for those with a solid attack strategy. When striving to achieve long-term fitness goals, maintaining faith in your ability to resolve any failure-and, there will be more than a few when faced with the daunting task of transforming your physique-is a vital necessity.

Approach your goals as if their realization were a foregone conclusion; realize in your heart that if things do not go precisely to plan, you will achieve all results and do not get discouraged. Most importantly, don't let anyone stop you from achieving good fat loss. Do not listen to those who are pessimistic, those who might even be delighted to see you fail. The biggest victory comes from demonstrating to yourself that anything of enduring value can be achieved. So, just listen to those who want to help you and ensure that you will accomplish all the obstacles that stand in your path.

FOUNDATION 10 YOUR DIET SUPPLEMENT

Regardless of how perfect your diet may seem, various nutritional deficiencies may compromise your results. It is wise to supplement with the quality of the soil used to grow much of our food that is deficient in life-giving minerals combined with different cooking techniques. Which also serves to destroy natural nutrients, along with the sheer volume of food needed to provide an adequate supply of certain nutrients. Supplementing is particularly essential for health and fitness because the training we do dictates special nutritional requirements that would be almost impossible to fulfill alone through a whole diet of foods.

Products such as white protein for muscle repair and glutamine are essential vitamins and minerals needed for proper cellular function and health maintenance. This serves the same purpose and enhances immune function, both of which are necessary, in my view, for optimal fat loss. Whey protein, being low in fat, allows one to replenish the protein stores rapidly without the excess calories that could be ingested from other sources. Although whole foods should remain the cornerstone of one's fat loss plan, it will increase one's chances of success by supplementing certain products.

For fat loss, the supplements I use and recommend are:

1. Protein Whey.
2. The Three Omega Fish Oils.
3. With glutamine.
4. A broad multi-vitamin and mineral product spectrum.
5. The extra vitamin C.

FOUNDATION 11 STAY MOTIVATED

Training success and one's level of motivation share a symbiotic relationship. High levels of motivation are required to achieve our training results, yet maintaining the motivation needed to continue to succeed often requires further success. One appears to be supporting the other. But we need a certain degree of motivation to start the training process first, and it will either gradually build or decline throughout one's training progression, depending on individual characteristics and various other factors, including, as mentioned, training success.

The objective here is to maintain high motivation levels during our body transformation - regardless of the degree of progress we achieve. It can be enormously stressful for the weight loss process. We will hit a plateau at a certain point in our program where the excess weight will fail to budge. This is precisely the moment when our motivation levels need to be strongest. One way to stay optimistic in such a situation is to evaluate what you have achieved and remember that progress can be attained. Speak to those who have faced similar challenges and issues and derive strength from them.

Ideally, you will be well served to read the numerous testimonials and tales of those who, against overwhelming odds, have found success in fat loss. You will read all of them right here on Bodybuilding.com. From several outlets, inspiration can be obtained. It can raise motivation levels by a kind comment or an encouraging word from a fellow gym member or the smallest improvements reported in your training log. Motivation and continuity underpin the success of fat loss, among all the pillars listed in this book.

FOUNDATION 12 IDENTIFYA TRAINING PARTNER

If you do not already have one, through the motivation they offer, a training partner can make a tremendous difference to the quality of your workouts-by encouraging you to push further than you may otherwise be motivated to-and the mutual goals they may have (they may face the same obstacles you do; by working together, both of you can find solutions

**Chapter 3: TIPS TO BUILDING A PLAN FOR LASTING
SUCCESS**

Gaining weight is not unusual. It's normal. However, if you
have realized that your weight gain is beyond what you think is
safe, then without having to make massive adjustments, there
are simple ways you can slim down easily. Better still, as long
as you incorporate any of the following strategies that truly
double down on your weight loss attempts, you will lose weight
in half the time.

Read on for 40 simple pointers that can shed those excess
pounds, and that can make your attempts to lose weight more
than twice as successful. And when you're done, check out
some extra tips that work for weight loss!

1.   Weighing up yourself

A two-year study conducted at Cornell University, according to
the Huffington Post, found that individuals who weighed
themselves regularly and reported those findings lost more
bodyweight and sustained fat loss better than those who did
not. Looking at the weight of your body also strengthens
weight loss ambitions and makes it harder to cheat on your
diet. The research illustrates how monitoring and tracking can
help rapid, permanent loss of fat, even doubling the amount of
weight you would otherwise lose without keeping track of it.
And see 20 Ways to Conquer a Weight Loss Plateau for more
ideas on weight loss.

2.   Do not Miss Food

That missing meal leads to weight loss is a common
misconception. Technically, you consume fewer calories at the
moment, but omitting a meal more often than not results in an
out-of-control appetite and irregular eating habits that are not
good for your metabolism. Simply put: It doesn't work to try to
minimize calories to lose weight. There are so many external

variables at stake. And see This Is the Perfect Time to Eat dinner, according to RDs, for a better understanding of timing your meals.

3. Eat a day of three healthy meals

Each of these three meals (plus a snack) should include flat-belly fat (olive oil, avocado) and a source of fiber, such as lentils, beans or quinoa, Power Protein (chicken, lean meat, fish, etc.). This will ensure a maximum loss of weight, partially because it will keep you full and discourage you from making poor decisions about food. And see 20 Fast & Simple Dinner Recipes for some balanced weeknight meal ideas.

4. Control the intake of sugar

You can point the finger at sugar, which has wormed its way through everything from tomato sauce to Advil caplets if you're looking for one thing to blame for those extra pounds. For optimum health, the American Heart Association and the World Health Organization advise no more than 25 grams of added sugar a day, around six sugar packets. Still, most individuals eat much more than that.

Keep INFORMED: To have the latest food news sent straight to your inbox, sign up for our email.

5. Add extra fiber to your diet

This vital nutrient makes you stay fuller longer, which means the more fiber you add into your diet, the less likely you will hit those chips or cookies in the mid-afternoon. If you are looking for a hassle-free way to easily shed pounds, reduce your intake of sugar, and consume more fiber than sugar. This easy adjustment to your diet will make you lose belly fat almost instantly and boot up fast. Want any thoughts? See 20 simple ways for your diet to add fiber.

6. Knowing How to Decipher a Food Label

It's very easy to take note of the calorie count and nothing else when you purchase processed food, but just because something is low in calories doesn't mean it'll be healthy in the long run for your waistline. Many low-calorie foods are filled with added sugar, which means they cause you to gain weight. When you want to lose weight, look for foods with more fiber than sugar. High-protein foods are also fantastic. Check out these 20 Tips for Actually Knowing Diet Labels for more expert advice.

7. Act Quickly

You'll see results in just a few days if you start the Zero Sugar Diet. And while we have been led to believe that rapid weight loss is potentially dangerous, according to a 2013 report in the International Journal of Behavioral Medicine. If you start from the gate by falling pounds quickly, you are more likely to succeed in your long-term weight loss goals. And see 40 Tips Nutritionists Tell You Must Follow to Lose Weight for more tips on falling pounds.

8. On the Protein Bag

Protein is also an essential component of a healthy diet, just like fiber, particularly if you're trying to lose weight. Research has shown that doubling your intake of protein will help you drop pounds without losing muscle mass, so make sure all your meals are high in protein and fiber but low in starch and sugar (think lean meat, fish, and soy). Here's what you need to hear on how to eat protein for optimum weight loss.

9. Know Your Combo Food

It's important to understand what food combinations will help your waistline continue to shrink once you've got the whole fiber/sugar balance down. For instance, cayenne powder and chicken pair well together because protein-rich foods can improve post-meal calorie burn dramatically, and chili peppers are great at blasting away belly fat. Bell peppers and eggs are another perfect combos. We smell your future with a veggie omelet!

10. Get Antioxidants for yourself

Antioxidants not only decrease the appearance of wrinkles and make you look younger, but they can also avoid the accumulation of fat. To double the weight loss, consume antioxidant-rich foods such as bananas, artichokes, and kidney beans (also high in fiber!).

11. Go Nuts For Nuts

Because of their high-calorie count, nuts get a bad reputation, but research shows that eating pistachios will accelerate weight loss instead of carb-based snacks. If consumed before a workout, almonds are equally helpful because they contain amino acids that help fry the belly fat—stock up on 6 of the Best Weight Loss Nuts.

12. Know the healthy fats

Eating fat to lose weight will sound counterintuitive, but you can improve your weight loss if you know which fats to eat. Eat foods rich in monounsaturated fat, such as avocado oil, macadamia nuts, and black or green olives, lose pounds. They're going to help fend off malnutrition and keep you lean!

13. Find the foods for you that work and stick to 'Em

There's something to be said about eating things you want over and over again, as David Zinczenko writes in Zero Sugar Diet, meaning you don't subsist on ice cream sundaes and chicken nuggets. As researchers looked at 6,814 people's diets, they found that the more varied one's diet was, the more likely one was to gain weight. Compared with those who had the least variety, those who consumed the widest range of foods showed a 120 percent greater increase in waist circumference. In other words, individuals who have the greatest weight loss results prefer a fixed number of foods and appear to stick to them. To lose weight, choose from these important foods!

14. Drink Responsibly

Mixed and/or cold beverages are usually filled with hundreds of empty calories, so opt instead for a glass of red or white wine if you're looking for a buzz. Just try to limit yourself to one glass of 5 ounces a day. Alcohol does, after all, have safe benefits!

15. Snack Smart

Believe it or not, it goes hand-in-hand with snacking and weight loss. Studies show that people who actively refrain from eating between meals, mostly because their energy reserves are low, can end up consuming more calories overall during the day, leading them to make poor choices. Make sure you do so responsibly when you are snacking. Like basic, air-popped popcorn and hummus, stick to high-fiber, high-protein treats. For more, check out the 50 best healthy snacks to buy for weight loss!

16. Use Smaller Dishes

Using smaller plates and bowls is a simple way to reduce your portion size and ensure you don't overeat, whether you're snacking or cooking a meal. Without feeling guilty, feel free to load up smaller dishes with fiber, protein, etc.

17. Get a Good Night Sleep

Dieters who sleep 5 minutes or less a night put on two and a half times more belly fat, according to Wake Forest researchers, while those who sleep more than eight hours put on only slightly less than that. Yet you set yourself up for day-in, day-out weight loss when you have a daily bedtime and stick to it. Look for six to seven hours of sleep a night, on average, the ideal amount for weight management. It could cut 200 calories a day by controlling your sleep schedule.

18. Understand the importance of strength training

Workouts for strength training contribute to solid muscles and provide many other advantages for fitness and weight loss. They also raise your level of energy, making it easier for daily tasks. And the more stamina you have, the more likely you are to keep busy with fast food instead of being parked in front of the TV.

19. Total Aerobic Exercises Interval-Training

Another perfect way to increase your fat-burning metabolism and boost your fitness without losing muscle is to do cardio workouts. But alternate brief bursts of quick, high-intensity exercise with bouts of slower, less-intensity "recovery" intervals instead of jumping on the treadmill and remaining at one speed. Many studies have shown that this form of exercise is highly successful for weight loss and belly fat targeting but avoid these 12 worst weight loss cardio mistakes.

20. No Cheating

"Cheat meals" are a popular gimmick used by many diet plans to help individuals cope with the difficulties of adhering to a strict diet schedule, but they break your momentum for weight loss and can even hurt your health. Researchers took blood samples from participants dealing with obesity and those who were lean and balanced in a 2015 research report in The FASEB Journal. Of instance, in terms of cholesterol and blood sugar, the samples showed different readings. Then, a high-calorie shake was offered to both classes. Those whose readings had been safe previously, when blood was taken from them after the shake, showed the same kind of increased risk factors for heart disease and diabetes as the unhealthy community.

21. Don't Watch TV Too Much

Overweight participants who cut their TV time by just 50 percent burned an additional 119 calories a day on average, a

University of Vermont study found. That's an annual twelve-pound automatic loss! Maximize these effects by multitasking as you watch, and your calorie burn will further bump up even light household activities. And if you're going to have a snack while watching TV, munch on the 7 Best Fat-Burning Foods.

22. Drink Ice Water with Ice

Dieting participants who were told to drink two cups of water before each meal lost 30 percent more weight than their thirsty peers in one University of Utah report. Part of the reason: If you don't drink enough water, you can store carbs as fat in your body. Without sufficient water, your body can not effectively change carbohydrates into energy. Apply ice to improve the calorie-burning effects of H2O. German researchers found that a metabolic boost that incinerates 50 extra daily calories could be triggered by six cups of cold water a day. You'll also want to see how much water for weight loss you need to drink.

23. Order at Restaurants First

Take care of your restaurant order if you want to take responsibility for your weight. A study from the University of Illinois found that groups of individuals tend to order similarly, especially when forced to say their order out loud. (Here's how you can eat and still lose weight at any restaurant.) In comparison, data from The New England Journal of Medicine suggests that when a friend becomes obese, it raises your risk of obesity by 57%.

24. Stress Eating Stop

Emotional eaters, those who acknowledged eating in reaction to emotional stress, were thirteen times more likely to be overweight or obese in a study by the University of Alabama. In response to stress, if you feel the urge to snack, consider chewing a piece of gum, chugging a glass of water, or walking around the block. Build an automated response that does not require food, and you can stop calorie overloading.

25. Get outside every morning

Sun exposure between 8:00 a.m. in studies Higher fat burning and slightly lower BMIs, regardless of exercise, calorie intake, sleep, or even age, are correlated with noon and noon. In the winter, one reason people appear to gain weight is that they're not out there as much. If it is hectic in the mornings, at least open the blinds in the morning, especially at work. During work hours, workers with windows above their desks gain 173 percent more exposure to white light and forty-six more minutes of sleep every night than workers who do not have natural light exposure. And less physical activity is provided to those without windows.

26. Using Grapefruit to eat

Grapefruit has an especially strong weight loss effect. A study published in the Metabolism journal found that eating half a grapefruit before meals can help lower visceral fat and lower levels of cholesterol. Six-week study participants who ate Rio Red grapefruit 15 minutes before breakfast, lunch, and dinner saw their waists shrink by as much as an inch, and LDL levels drop by 18 points. The results are due by researchers to a mixture of phytochemicals and vitamin C in the grapefruit. Check out these 20 Weight Loss Grapefruit Recipes here.

27. Embrace casual business

Casual wear, as opposed to traditional business dress, will increase physical activity levels in our daily routines, a report by the American Council on Exercise suggests. The study participants took an additional 491 steps and burned 25 more calories, wearing jeans on days compared to conventional suit wear. This may sound trivial, but the calories are adding up! Researchers estimate that keeping it informal only once a week could eliminate 6,250 calories over the year, enough to counteract most Americans' average annual weight gain (0.4 to 1.8 pounds).

28. Leave Yourself Motivating Notes

A 2015 study in the Journal of Marketing Research found that if you're trying to lose weight, subtle, even subliminal, messages can be more effective in helping you adhere to a healthy eating routine than even constant, conscious concentration. The study showed that people who receive reinforcing notes urging them to eat healthily are more likely to make smarter decisions than those who have only tried to keep their goals top of mind.

29. Tell No to the Basket of Bread

Dining out when dieting is difficult, but turning down the beginning of the meal bread basket is one way to ensure you stay on track. At some restaurants, breadsticks, cookies, and chips and salsa can be complimentary, but that does not mean you're not going to pay for them. Each time you eat one of the free breadsticks from Olive Garden or Cheddar Bay Biscuits from Red Lobster, you add 150 calories to your meal. Over dinner, eat three, and that's 450 calories. That's also approximately the amount of calories you can expect at your favorite Mexican restaurant for every basket of tortilla chips you get. And the twenty best and worst store-bought bread are here.

30. Between bites, put your fork down

It takes your stomach twenty minutes to convince your brain that you have enough, which means it can be difficult to pinpoint exactly when you are finished. Research in the Journal of the American Dietetic Association showed that slow eaters consumed 66 fewer calories per meal. Still, they felt like they had eaten more relative to their fast-eating peers. What, you wonder, is 66 calories? You can lose more than twenty pounds a year if you can do that at every meal! An easy trick to slow your pace: After each slice, simply put your fork down on the plate.

31. Keep away from meals with combos and value

"A report in the Journal of Public Policy & Marketing shows

that by going for the" combo "or" value meal, "you pick up a hundred or more extra calories compared to ordering à la carte." Why? Why? And you're likely to buy more food than you want when you order things bundled together. You're best off buying your piecemeal food and going for The 100 Healthiest Foods on the Planet when you do.

32. Don't Drive to work

According to a report in the British Medical Journal, those who drive to work gain more weight than those who use public transportation. Commuting by car slaps an additional 5.5 pounds on your body, whether you workout or not, according to the report.

33. Walkthrough the Office

We sit sixty-seven hours a week on average, sitting nine hours a day, eight hours lying down, and just about seven hours out of every twenty-four hours spent actively moving. Today, our sedentary occupations cause us to burn 100 fewer calories a day compared to 50 years ago. That alone means gaining an additional ten pounds a year. But a recent study in the American Society of Nephrology's Clinical Journal found that taking a two-minute stroll every hour might mitigate the effects of too much sitting. Make it a habit never to call a colleague when you can stop talking just as easily at his or her office. See more ways in which you can lose weight at work!

34. Leave Work on Time

Add work hours at the beginning of the day, not the end, when deadlines pile up. You also eat more and go to sleep later as you work later, all of which add to unnecessary pounds. Those whose last meal was nearest to bedtime took in more calories overall during the day than those who allowed their bodies time to rest before going to bed, a report in the journal Nutrition Research showed.

35. Stick to Wet Carbs

Modern nutrition gurus have made carbs look so frightening, but new research shows that when you keep guessing, your fat-burning method actually works better, so don't let yourself get stuck in a rut. According to the journal Basics of Strength Training and Conditioning, eating a range of carbohydrates is also desirable, at least for athletes. Bear in mind; this is no invitation to the Froot Loops gorge. Try focusing more on "wet" carbs, especially at night, instead. A wet carb, like cucumbers, onions, salad greens, and asparagus, is one that naturally has a lot of water in it. Since you can't drink while you sleep, wet carbs help you to maintain adequate water levels during the night. Staying hydrated overnight means that even though you're dreaming of a faraway cove, your body can continue to get the nourishment it needs to expose your abs. Here are 11 more eating habits that your abs will reveal!

36. Stop Eating Family-Style

Do you know how dinner with a lovely composition and a little sprig of parsley on the side is served in a fancy restaurant? Instead of just throwing everything on a platter and putting it out for the rabble to reach for, do it at home. Research in the Obesity journal showed that when family-style food is served, individuals eat 35 percent more throughout the meal. When leaving the table needs additional support, people hesitate to go back for more.

37. Drink some tea

Strong weight loss drinks are coffee and tea in particular. What's more there? For various purposes, various varieties of tea cause you to lose weight. For instance, green tea acts as a metabolism booster because it activates your fat cells, while white tea prevents new fat cells. Keep away from sweeteners and just opt to have a squeeze of lemon in your tea. Lemon will potentially boost the weight-loss powers of the beverage. Read more about the Five Best Weight Loss Teas!

38. Avoid Artificial Sweeteners

We said you're not supposed to put artificial sweeteners in your tea, and if we're truthful, they don't have a place in your diet anywhere else, either, particularly if you're trying to lose weight. Artificial sweeteners produce belly fat and lead us to reach for extra calories, not to mention havoc on the health of your teeth, heart, and stomach.

39. Tamp Down Your Dreams

It's okay to dream big, but you may be better off dreaming about yourself getting big when it comes to weight loss. A study in the Cognitive Therapy and Research journal found that obese women who fantasized about weight loss and showing off their hot new bodies lost an average of twenty-four pounds less than those who had negative thoughts, such as how awful they might look if they continued to eat poorly. The researchers hypothesized that the dieters were prepared by pessimistic fantasies about weight loss to conquering the bumps they experienced on their way to getting well.

40. Become Autonomous

A 2012 study throughout the International Journal of Behavioral Nutrition and Physical Activity found that you are more likely to see long-lasting health improvements if you feel independent; in other words, you have complete control and don't need to rely on a diet plan. And for more information on weight loss, see The Weight Loss Best & Worst Diets.

10 TRICKS FOR SEEING WEIGHT LOSS FAST RESULTS

Slow and steady wins the race when it comes to losing pounds. While fad diets can lead to rapid weight loss, these restrictive plans are difficult to stick with, and once you slip off the wagon, the weight eventually creeps back. As you have learned time and time again, it takes a permanent lifestyle change to reach weight loss that you can sustain.

This is always better said than achieved. It can be a challenge to stick to a healthy diet and exercise regimen, particularly if you do not see the positive results you are looking for in a relatively short period. We consulted the health experts for some of their best tricks to get and see to keep you inspired and working towards your target! Results rapidly. These tried-and-true tips will inspire you to stick with it, whether you have five or 50 pounds to lose.

Weigh Yourself on Friday

Studies have shown that individuals who frequently weigh themselves are more effective in losing weight and keeping it off. When is the most appropriate time to weigh in? On Fridays and Mondays, I encourage my clients to get on the scale. During the week, individuals prefer to adhere to their good routines and loosen the reins somewhat on the weekend. During the week, weighing in on Friday will demonstrate the outcomes of your hard work and allow you to take the practices into the weekend. Your Monday weigh-in may show a few extra pounds and inspire you to get right back on track if you've indulged over the weekend. Throughout the week, keep a graph to document weight fluctuation trends, which will help you make a better diet and exercise decisions to achieve your goals.

Eat Off of Appetizer Plates

Over the years, plate sizes have shifted, rising in diameter, much like our waistlines. Dinner plates from our great grandmother looked like today's salad plates. We are all visual, and when we eat on smaller plates, it's so much easier to eat the correct portion and feel fulfilled, "says Cheryl Harris, MPH, RD, Virginia's holistic eating coach." Try ordering your salad or appetizer and sharing a main dish if you're dining in a restaurant that uses plates the size of manhole covers. Ask the waiter to wrap half your dish in a doggy bag while dining out alone before it is served, and enjoy the rest on a smaller appetizer plate. You will never know what you're missing!

Add fat or sugar to your salad

Salads are a nutritional no-brainer when adopting a healthy-eating plan. But while a good option for weight loss is to load up on non-starchy vegetables, it can also leave you feeling deprived, leading to later binge-eating. Add a crunchy, creamy, or sweet ingredient, including nuts and seeds, avocado, or dried fruit, to keep salads satisfying. And make sure you cover the salad with a protein filling, such as grilled chicken or fish.

Water to drink before every meal

Before you sit down to eat, reaching for a bottle of water may help you shed those pounds faster. A study in the August 2015 Obesity Journal showed that obese patients lost almost 3 pounds more than those who did not drink 500 milliliters (a 16-ounce bottle) of water 30 minutes before feeding. Perhaps more surprising is that over 12 weeks (compared to a 2-pound weight loss for those who preloaded before only one meal, or not at all), those pre-loaded with water before each of the three main meals lost an average of 10 pounds.

Vanessa Stasio Costa, RDN, a diet consultant in New York City, says that sipping on water during the day "helps to stop overeating caused by mistaking the thirst signal for hunger." By adding flavored ice cubes, or fruit slices and herbs, you can keep the water interesting.

Add Biceps Curls to Your Routine

To get in shape, you do not have to attend an expensive fitness club or spend hours in the gym. It can have a big effect on how you look and feel by simply incorporating some strength-training exercises to your routines, such as biceps curls and pushups. "You're going to feel better a few weeks in, long before you start seeing results," says Caroline Kaufman, MS, RDN, a Los Angeles diet consultant. "It's going to be easier to bring food, or you'll be able to throw the big suitcase like a pro into the overhead bin." These exercises are easy to do, can be performed in the comfort of your own home, and if you have a few spare minutes, it can be squeezed into your schedule. These physical improvements will keep you inspired as you develop muscles, become more toned, and lose inches.

Clutch at parties with your purse and a glass of water

Lorraine Matthews-Antosiewicz, MS, RD, a food and nutrition expert in New Jersey, suggests that if you tend to overeat at cocktail parties, "choose a non-caloric beverage when you first arrive and delay eating anything until you have a chance to look over all the choices." You can determine which indulgent treats you want to splurge on by scoping out what's available and which lean, filler foods will help fill you up. Keeping in one hand a low-calorie soda and in the other, a pocket will keep you from grazing mindlessly. Matthews-Antosiewicz says, "Choose one or two hors d'oeuvres that you want and then wait until the cocktail hour is almost over before placing them on your plate, especially if there is a meal to follow." To fill your plate, you will have to set down what you are holding, which will keep you mindful of what and how much you are eating.

After-slice put your fork down!

It allows you to eat less by savoring each bite of food and paying attention to flavor, texture, and temperature, so you will be more in tune with your levels of hunger and satisfaction. "Simply placing your utensil between food bites could stop you from 'shoveling in' more mindlessly than you need," says Sara Haas, RD, and chef. Haas recommends that when you chew, you take a bite and then let your fork relax next to your plate. Mindful eating allows time for the body to show that you are full and helps digestion.

Hide Treats in the Garage

Although treats such as chocolate, candy, and cookies may look lovely in clear glass jars on your countertop, having them front and center will make them a constant temptation. "Julie Upton, MS, RD, blogger at Appetite for Fitness, suggests" Keep [treats] in very awkward locations, such as in your shed or hard-to-access parts of your kitchen. "Cover them with aluminum foil if you have them in your refrigerator or pantry, so you can't see the food and won't be as tempted by it."

Have your dessert ready before you head out for dinner

The minute you see the fudgy chocolate cake delivered to the table next to you, all your good thoughts go out the door, you tell yourself you're not going to order dessert. Abbey Sharp, RD, a nutrition expert in Toronto, suggests keeping a treat waiting at home to help you protect against temptations. "Put aside a portion-controlled sweet for yourself at home before you go out to eat, like a tiny cookie or a square of melted dark chocolate with fresh berries," Sharp says. Or try cooking up a dessert like a light angel food cake with fresh berries for the whole family, which will give everyone something to look forward to.

Count to 10 between the first three bites of your

Focusing on the taste of food instead of the thing you are doing when eating (like looking at a TV screen or reading emails) is another trick to promote mindful eating. "By concentrating on the first three to six bites of food, cultivate[you're] taste buds," says Chere Bork, MS, RD, a Minneapolis speaker, and wellness coach. Taste buds are chemical receptors that get exhausted very easily, so the first few bites of a meal will taste better than the next few bites unless you are very hungry. You will have very little taste experience after a larger amount. By savoring the early bites, particularly when it comes to rich foods such as chocolate and cheese, you will satisfy hunger and cravings without consuming large p p.

Chapter 4: BUILDING A GOOD RELATIONSHIP WITH FOOD

Many individuals feel that healthy eating is entirely about what you put on your plate. People are focused on the merits of these micronutrients, macros, probiotics, and avoiding items like GMOs and non-organic products. But what does or does not go on your fork is not one of the most critical aspects of healthy eating; it maintains a healthy food relationship.

Many individuals have a complex relationship with food, partially because of the very vocabulary we use to speak about how we eat. Many foods come with an implied "positive" or "poor" correlation created by our own expectations and society's standards, such as calling junk food (a "poor") chips and desserts versus other highly nutrient-dense foods called superfoods (a "positive)."

This may not sound like a big deal, but the language can affect how we feel about ourselves for eating or even choosing to eat those foods. "A lot of people pass these labels into their self-worth; if I eat 'healthy' food, I am good. If I eat ' bad 'food, I am bad, " says Camille Williams, MA, LCPC, the eating disorder program leader at treatment center Timberline Knolls.

This kind of black-and-white thinking can generate embarrassment and guilt — which in turn influences how and what you eat. "Categorizing foods as 'good' or 'bad' can induce some mental restraint, where we feel poorly after consuming 'bad foods' and then tell ourselves we'll never eat that way again. Alissa Rumsey, MS, RD, a licensed intuitive consuming counselor, and owner of Alissa Rumsey Nutrition and Wellness, previously told Well+Good. It can build a loop where you restrict food, gorge on certain foods, feel bad about it, then work to restrict again. It's unhealthy for physical and mental health — and can potentially lead to disordered eating patterns.

The truth, of course, is that at any single point in your life, eating a donut or a bowl of mac and cheese or any kind of food does not make you a bad person or even an overweight person. But it is complicated and takes time to untangle a destructive relationship with food. To be healthier, happier, and guilt-free, Williams and Rumsey share ways to start reframing your relationship with your food.

Food. You can't live with it sometimes, and you certainly can't live without it. Most of us have some food or macronutrient issues, and that's why we're forced to work on our food relationships over and over again. All the conflicting or one-sided dietary knowledge that often pops up is what makes things much more difficult. You know the drill, carbs are evil, meat is murder, good fats vs. bad fats. With a lot of noise and nothing to eat, we're left.

Experts will continue to disagree, and there will always be new research emerging. In the end, maintaining a healthy food relationship means learning to turn the volume down, loosen the rules, and avoid setting yourself up for failure.

I am a nutritionist and fitness coach who is holistic. Here's my take on how to have a balanced eating relationship.

With rules, be careful

It is no wonder that orthorexia is on the rise. Structure and guidelines allow us to feel protected from overindulgent food guilt; an obsession with consuming foods that one considers good, while systematically avoiding foods that are perceived to be unhealthy. Not to mention, from our ability to show regulation and obey the food rules we build for ourselves, we experience a surge of trust. But the knee-jerk reaction when we falter is to tighten the reins, eventually setting ourselves up for failure. Plus, for micronutrient imbalances and deficiencies in the body, you can set up unattainable controls.

Don't get ready for failure

It doesn't matter whether you're a CEO, an actress, an artist, or an accountant, you were raised to celebrate with a cake around a table, which is perfect as an occasional treat. It's the person you are. It's a stretch to buy candy favorites in bulk and expect 100 percent to be under control beyond a short-term, 30-day reset cleanse. Sugar is a key to choices and remorse over unhealthy eating. Step out for a single-serving, protein-packed, gluten-free cookie instead of stocking this medication in your kitchen or keep your homemade coconut oil freezer fudge on hand.

Avoid appeasing your mate

If gluten does not make you feel healthy, don't eat it. To show the milk doesn't work for you, you don't need a blood test. Trust your intuition. Go for it if you want to be a vegetarian. I'm impressed when you're a Paleo CrossFitter. Let's all make a promise to stop eating for others, stop criticizing their decisions, and focus on what we need. If that means missing a course at a dinner party with your mate, so be it and do so guilt-free.

Yeah, be careful to remove food and build guidelines, but don't make excuses, clarify the choices that make you feel good, or defend them. And be ready to improve your eating habits (which is another excuse to stop preaching about them).

Nourishment Priority

Food can harm you, but it can heal you as well. Wild proteins, natural fats, and leafy greens can help you bear an infant, heal injuries, develop shiny hair, and create powerful muscles. Avoiding refined foods and excessive sugar will make you feel bright, sleep soundly, and evade food-related illnesses, including diabetes, metabolic syndrome, and heart disease.

But if you concentrate on what you can't consume, you expend your mental energy in a room that fuels the fire of desire. Unwind. Relax. Take one meal at a time, and I promise you're not going to starve. "Simply sit down and ask yourself the question," What for the next few hours will nourish and sustain me?

Reflect on what to eat, not what to avoid

At-meal, if you eat protein, fat, and fibrous greens, you are guaranteed to fill up on what your body needs and remain full for longer. When you are satisfied, you won't be drooling over a cupcake left in the office kitchen. At lunch, without dressing, a chicken salad on iceberg lettuce is not going to do it. Instead, to make it last until a late snack or dinner, add avocado or nuts.

For breakfast, the same goes; don't skimp. Then expect to overeat or cave in the afternoon if you are counting calories in the morning. Fill up on protein and fat early instead. This has been shown to satisfy you, stretch your blood sugar curve, and help you eat less in general.

The beWELL Smoothie is the method my clients use to keep calm until the early afternoon. They should up their consumption of fat, fiber, or protein as needed to peacefully head into lunch. When you aren't hungry, you make better choices and meals. Instead of counting calories and attempting to consume less, focus on consuming the food that will turn off hunger signals the longest.

Remember: Balance Isn't About Perfection

Be Well; we aim to instill equilibrium in our clients. Bingeing and cleansing periods swing you back and forth like an out-of-control pendulum. Happiness and health are achieved when you achieve equilibrium. Contrary to common opinion, equilibrium isn't when you stop moving and live a static, scheduled, and " perfect " life. None of us is fine. You can bounce a little from time to time. We all do. Balance is sought through deliberate movement to eat clean, sweat, and even enjoy a glass of wine through friends.

Accept who you are, enjoy who you are, and develop a lifestyle based on health, not some vague notion of " perfection. "Punishing yourself for" failing "is unhealthy, unproductive, and breeds disappointment. By concentrating on consuming whole, nutrient-dense food, and trying to develop a balanced, active lifestyle, you'll take the essential first steps to be well.

ADDITIONAL TIPS FOR MAINTAINING AN HEALTHY RELATIONSHIP WITH FOOD

Some people eat emotionally, which is detrimental to maintaining a healthy lifestyle and losing unwanted pounds, to isolate themselves from their emotions. Because they are stressed, sad, bored, or lonely, people sometimes eat. Typically, people who eat emotionally reach for unhealthy "comfort food," such as french fries or ice cream, leading to obesity, diabetes, and heart disease.

Some people are addicted to food, often unhealthy things like chocolate, pizza, and chips for snacks. "Clifford says," Some people [are compulsive] about food, the same way some people are about alcohol or gambling. "Parallels exist."

But there is a food compulsion that differs from other conditions. For alcoholism and gambling, there are rehab centers and 12-step programs, but everyone needs to eat.

Experts offer these tips to achieve and maintain healthy eating habits and prevent food from becoming an opponent or a too-close friend:

1. Don't label good or bad for specific foods. There are no angelic health powers in a cup of broccoli, and a slice of pizza is not demonic. Some foods are better than others for your well-being, but no food is either evil or benevolent, says Anne Lewis, an Indianapolis clinical psychologist at Indiana University Health.

Lewis says that ascribing moral qualities to foods gives them unwarranted power. If you deviate from your diet and eat fast food, it doesn't make you a bad person, and you needn't beat yourself up for it, which might lead to a feeling of defeat and overeating. Maintain a balanced outlook on food by recognizing that certain foods are better for your health than others, but no particular form of food or portion can ensure or destroy your well-being.

2. Minimize the motivation to make poor decisions. It's OK to have a small slice of cake on special occasions, such as your birthday or when you're out having dinner with friends, Lewis says, if you're on a low-sugar diet.

Limit the intake of your cake to rare cases. Lewis says that having some foods nearby will foster a habit of consuming them, not having cake in the house. Give it away or throw it out if you have a birthday party at your home and have leftover cake.

3. Don't get too restrictive. Instead of fully cutting out those foods, encourage yourself to have a moderate portion of your favorite treat one day a week. Instead of trying to banish donuts from your diet forever, for instance, give yourself one every seven days, says Clifford.

It may be impractical to try not to consume a single food for the rest of your life. Instead of feeling like a failure if you have that food, which may result in more binge eating, integrate that food in moderation into your eating routine.

4. Keep your food diary. Write down not only what you're eating, but what you feel at the moment. Clifford advises that documenting your eating habits and emotions will assist you in detecting patterns.

You might see that you backslide from your good eating habits by consuming chips, cookies, and other junk foods when you're feeling sad, anxious, or depressed. Rather than trying to reach for the unhealthy snack, try doing some deep breathing or going for a short walk. "If you try that, instead, the craving will pass a lot of times," Clifford says.

5. Just try cooking. Take the time to cook instead of eating your meal in a microwave or picking up your food on the way home from a deli or fast-food joint. Make a list of delicious and healthy ingredients from the store that you need and enjoy choosing them.

You don't have to become a master chef. "Cooking can be very simple," says Clifford. You can buy a steamer and toss it with your vegetables. Good indoor grills are available. If you go to the store to pick and prepare your ingredients, you appreciate your food more. It makes you mindful of it.'

6. At the grocery store, set yourself up for success. Dr. Michael Russo, a general surgeon, specializing in bariatric surgery at the MemorialCare Center for Obesity at Orange Coast Memorial Medical Center in Fountain Valley, California, says that the battle to maintain a balanced relationship with food begins at the supermarket, where what you buy will greatly determine whether you will maintain healthy eating habits.

To avoid aisles loaded with unhealthy items, your shopping trips can be strategized. "With cookies, crackers, snack chips, and other processed or refined foods high in carbohydrates, the last thing you want to do is load up your cart," Russo says. We are facing an obesity epidemic for the single most important reason. "Try shopping only at the perimeter of the supermarket, where fresh produce, lean meats, milk products, and baked products are sold, and avoid inside aisles, where snack items and sugar desserts are usually sold, Russo says." They are the single most important reason why we face an obesity epidemic. Pick whole-grain bread and avoid cakes, muffins, and cookies when you are in the bakery section.

Chapter 5: EXPLORING THE MIND BODY CONNECTION WITH HYPNOSIS

Mind-body medicine is on the verge of changing modern healthcare. During the last thirty years, scientists have started to investigate the interconnections between mind and body and how these are connected to our inherent healing capabilities. As this development occurs, mind-body modalities will secure their place among the many complementary-alternative treatments that can be beneficial for health maintenance and healing.

Hypnosis delves into the darkest phases of the mind using the power of suggestion and trance states. The result: modified behavioral habits and treatment influence a wide variety of health conditions. Up to fifteen thousand doctors are currently integrating hypnotherapy with conventional medical treatments. Hypnotherapy is estimated to help 94 percent of patients, but it is only linked to increased relaxation.

Hypnosis can support many psychological and physical conditions, including habit regulation. Behavior change for nail-biting, smoking, stuttering), weight management (reprogramming eating habits), pain control (e.g., back pain, arthritis, chronic pain, migraine), stress and anxiety reduction (reduce stress and help keep life events in perspective), phobia removal (e.g., reduce common fears), imagination (remove blocked potential), goal-setting (set and accomplish attainable goals), sleep recovery (improve sleep onset and sound sleep), and motivation (increase confidence). It is also used for various other health issues, including stomach disorders, respiratory conditions, anxiety, and certain dental-related problems such as anxiety or as part of a pain-management plan.

Early Hypnosis References to hypnosis have existed for thousands of years. Ancient literature, myths, and scriptural texts include mention of consciousness and primitive forms of hypnosis. From the scientific viewpoint, an early reference to altered states and the power to magnetic fields dates back to the time of Swiss physician Paracelsus (1493-1541) and later, to Swiss mesmerist Charles Lafontaine and Austrian theorist, Dr. Franz Anton Hypnotic (1733 -1815).

Nevertheless, the title,' Father of Hypnosis,' belongs to Dr. James Braid, MRCS (1795-1860), an English physician. Even though medical authorities initially rejected hypnosis, Braid eventually made it a respectable medical practice. The successful results of Braid eventually attracted Sigmund Freud's attention and C.J. Jung, both of whom explored its uses as a therapeutic instrument briefly.

Clark Hull (1884-1952) helped move hypnosis into the realm of psychology in 1933. The British Medical Society officially recognized modern Hypnosis Hypnosis in 1955 as a legitimate medical procedure, and the American Medical Association and the American Psychological Association followed suit in 1958.

The influence of the American psychiatrist, Milton H. Erikson (1901-1980) came with advancement and acceptance. Erikson believed that within us, we all have the resources required for change. By providing the client with options, it is the hypnotherapist that helps the client to awaken these latent potentials. As a result of this view, hypnosis is considered by many professionals to be the induction (application) of a naturally occurring trance state.

Hypnosis versus hypnotherapy After treating more than 30,000 hypnosis patients, Erikson tried to differentiate between hypnosis and hypnotherapy. The process that follows hypnosis is seen as hypnotherapy. Many hypnotists are, therefore, not hypnotherapists. The distinction between the two types of professionals is made by training in mental health. Stage hypnosis is neither therapeutic hypnosis nor hypnotherapy and is performed for entertainment purposes.

Depending on the technique and the personal psychology of

the clients, clients may experience hypnosis differently. Some individuals experience intense awareness, others deep relaxation. The hypnotist's instructional words may be clear, but barely audible at other times. The voice of the hypnotist may seem to fade in and out for some individuals. Eriksonian research showed that the client is always free to change the hypnotic experience and come at will out of the trance.

What is hypnotherapy?

Hypnosis is a technique several clinicians use to help people achieve a state of complete relaxation. During a session, therapists assume that the conscious and unconscious mind can focus and concentrate on verbal repetition and mental imagery. The subconscious, as a result, becomes open to suggestions and open to change concerning attitudes, feelings, and habits.

Since the 1700s, variants of this holistic treatment have helped individuals with everything from bed-wetting to nail-biting to smoking. Research on hypnosis has also shown some potential for treating obesity, as we'll discuss in this book.

Does hypnotherapy work for weight loss?

Hypnosis can be more successful than diet and exercise alone for people trying to lose weight. The theory is that the subconscious can be conditioned to alter behaviors like overeating. However, just how successful it might be is still up for discussion.

One earlier controlled trial investigated the use of hypnotherapy for weight loss in people with obstructive sleep apnea. The research looked at two unique types of hypnotherapy against simple diet recommendations for weight loss and sleep apnea. Both 60 participants lost 2 to 3 percent of their body weight in 3 months.

At the 18-month follow-up, the hypnotherapy participant had lost another 8 pounds on average. The researchers concluded that although this additional loss wasn't major, hypnotherapy needed further study to treat obesity.

A study that included hypnotherapy for weight loss, specifically cognitive behavioral therapy (CBT), found that it resulted in a slight decrease in body weight relative to the placebo community. Researchers concluded that while hypnotherapy may boost weight loss, there is not enough research to be conclusive.

In favor of hypnosis alone for weight loss, it is important to remember that there is not much research. Most of what you'll think, in conjunction with diet and exercise or counseling, is about hypnotherapy.

What Is Weight Loss Hypnosis?

You already hear about the regular go-to providers when it comes to losing weight: doctors, nutritionists, and dietitians, personal trainers, also mental health coaches. But there might be one that you haven't talked of quite yet: a hypnotist.

Using hypnosis, it turns out, is another path people venture down in the name of weight loss. And usually, after all the other last-ditch attempts (I see you, juice cleanses and fad diets) are attempted and failed, it's traveled, says Greg Gurniak, a licensed Ontario clinical and medical hypnotist.

But it's not about someone else manipulating your mind and making you do humorous stuff when you're unconscious. "Mind regulation and losing control—aka doing something against your will—are the greatest myths regarding hypnosis," says Kimberly Friedmutter, hypnotherapist and author of Subconscious Power: Use Your Inner Mind to Build the Existence You've Always Desired. "Because of how the film industry depicts hypnotists, people are pleased to see I'm not wearing a black robe and spinning a watch from a chain."

You're still not unconscious when you undergo hypnosis — it's more of a deep state of relaxation, Friedmutter says. "It's the normal, floaty feeling you get before you drift off to sleep or the dreamy sensation you get when you wake up in the morning before you're completely conscious of where you are and what is around you."

Being in that state makes you more prone to change, and that's why hypnosis for weight loss can be successful. "It's different from other approaches because hypnosis examines the cause and other contributing factors directly at the subconscious level of the person's mind, where their memories, behaviors, worries, food associations, negative self-talk, and self-esteem germinate," says Capri Cruz, Ph.D., psychotherapist, and hypnotherapist and author of Enhance The Super Powers. "No other weight loss tool tackles the key problems at the root as hypnosis does."

There is not much recent, randomized research available on the subject, but what is out there indicates that the technique may be plausible. Early research in the 1990s showed that those who used hypnosis lost more than twice as much weight without cognitive therapy as those who died. Research published in 2014 worked with 60 obese women and found that those who practiced hypnobehavioral therapy lost weight and improved their eating patterns and body image. And a small 2017 study operated with eight obese adults and three kids, all of whom successfully lost weight, with one even rejecting surgery due to the benefits of treatment, but none of that, of course, is conclusive.

"The unfortunate factor is that medical insurance is not readily provided by hypnosis, so there is not the same push for hypnosis trials as there is for pharmaceutical ones," says Dr. Cruz. But with the seemingly ever-increasing cost of prescription medications, lengthy lists of potential side effects, and the drive for more natural alternatives, Cruz is optimistic that as a feasible solution to weight loss, hypnosis will soon gain more exposure and testing.

For weight loss, who can try hypnosis?

Anyone who has difficulty sticking to a balanced diet and exercise regimen is, frankly, the perfect candidate because they do not seem to shake their bad habits, Gurniak says. It is a sign of a subconscious issue to get trapped in unhealthy patterns, like eating the whole bag of potato chips instead of stopping when you're finished, he says.

Your subconscious, Friedmutter states, is where your thoughts, behaviors, and addictions are located. And it could be more powerful because hypnotherapy tackles the subconscious rather than just the aware. A 1970 study review found that hypnosis had a success rate of 93 percent, with fewer sessions required than both psychotherapy and behavioral therapy. "This led researchers to conclude that hypnosis was the most powerful tool for modifying attitudes, thought patterns, and actions," Friedmutter says.

However, hypnotherapy doesn't have to be used alone. Gurniak says that hypnosis can also be used to treat various health conditions, be it diabetes, obesity, arthritis, or cardiovascular disease, as a supplement to other weight loss programs developed by clinicians.

What should I expect during a treatment?

Sessions can differ in duration and technique, depending on the practitioner. Dr. Cruz, for example, says her sessions usually last between 45 and 60 minutes, while Friedmutter sees weight loss patients for three to four hours. But in general, you can expect to lie back, relax with your eyes closed, and let the hypnotherapist direct you through practical strategies and ideas that can help you achieve your goals.

"The concept is to train the mind to shift toward what is good and away from what is unhealthy," Friedmutter says. "Through client background, I can establish subconscious hitches that sent the client off their original blueprint of [health]. Just as we learn to abuse our bodies with food, we should learn to respect them.

And no, you won't be clucking like a chicken or confessing some deep, dark secrets. "You cannot be trapped in hypnosis or forced to say or do anything against your will," Gurniak says. "If it goes against your principles or convictions, you obviously will not act on the knowledge being given during trance."

Instead, you may feel a deep relaxation, while still being mindful of what's being said, Gurniak says. "Someone in a hypnotic trance would characterize it as in between being wide awake and asleep, " he says. "They are completely in charge and able to interrupt the process at any moment, since you can only be hypnotized if you want to. We function as a team to achieve the purpose of the individual.

During hypnotherapy, your counselor will likely begin your session by describing how hypnosis works. They'll then go over the personal goals. From there, your therapist can begin speaking in a calming, gentle voice to help you relax and create a feeling of protection.

When you've reached a more receptive state of mind, your therapist might recommend ways to help you change your eating or exercise habits or other ways to achieve your weight loss goals.

Certain words or repetition of certain phrases can help with this point. Your therapist can also help you imagine yourself achieving goals by sharing vivid mental imagery.

To close the session, the therapist will help get you out of hypnosis and back to the starting state.

The length of the hypnosis session and the number of total sessions you will need will depend on your objectives. Some people can see results in as little as one to three sessions.

Forms of hypnotherapy

There are various forms of hypnotherapy. Suggestion therapy

is most widely used for behaviors like smoking, nail-biting, and eating disorders.

Your therapist can also use hypnotherapy along with other therapies, including diet advice or CBT.

Hypnotherapy costs

The cost of hypnotherapy varies depending on where you live and the therapist you select. Consider calling ahead to negotiate rates or sliding scale options.

Your insurance company may cover between 50 and 80 percent of therapy offered by licensed professionals. Again, call ahead to learn more about your particular coverage.

You will find licensed therapists by asking your primary doctor for a referral or by searching the American Society for Clinical Hypnosis database of providers.

Benefits of hypnotherapy

The biggest advantage of hypnosis is that it helps people to reach a comfortable state of mind where they could be more open to advise to help improve their behaviors. For others, this can mean quicker and more prominent performance — but this isn't true for all.

Studies suggest that certain individuals may be more sensitive to the effects of hypnosis and, therefore, more likely to benefit from it. Certain personality traits may make a person more susceptible to hypnosis, such as selflessness and openness.

Studies have found that sensitivity to hypnosis rises after age 40, and women, regardless of age, are more likely to be responsive.

Hypnosis is considered effective for most people if done under the guidance of a professional practitioner. It isn't a means for brainwashing or mind control. A therapist can't manipulate a person to the point of doing something humiliating or something against their will.

Hypnotherapy risks

Again, for most individuals, hypnosis is healthy. It is unusual to have adverse reactions.

Main risks include:

- Headache
- Dizziness
- Drowsiness
- Anxiety
- Distress
- False memory creation

Before attempting hypnotherapy, people who encounter hallucinations or delusions can talk to their psychiatrist. Also, hypnosis under the influence of drugs or alcohol should not be done on a person.

Additional weight loss tips

To support your weight loss efforts, here are some things you can do at home:

Most days of the week, move your body. Try to get 150 minutes of moderate activity a week (such as cycling, water aerobics, gardening) or 75 minutes of more intensive exercise (such as running, swimming laps, climbing hills).

Maintain a journal of food. Track how much you eat, what you eat, and whether you're eating out of hunger or not. Doing so will help you determine patterns to modify, such as snacking out of boredom.

Eat vegetables and berries. Per day, strive for five servings of fruit and vegetables. To reduce your appetite, you can also add more fiber to your diet, about 25 to 30 grams per day.

Drink six to eight glasses a day of water. Being moisturized helps reduce overeating.

Withstand the temptation to miss meals. Eating all day long helps to keep your metabolism running high.

While hypnosis may provide an advantage over other methods of weight loss, it's not always a fast fix. Even so, research does indicate that it may benefit from using it in tandem with a healthy diet, physical exercise, and other therapies.

To assess the use of hypnosis for more substantial weight loss, more research is needed. Consider asking your doctor for a referral to a nutritionist or other specialist for additional support, who can help you develop an individual weight loss plan to achieve your goals.

Chapter 6: UNDERSTANDING THE POWER OF BELIEF IN WEIGHT LOSS

Where do you want this to go?

When we start a weight loss journey, we have preconceived assumptions about how it will go. Popular ones are that it will be hard, that it will take deprivation, that you may not be able to do it, or that you aren't sure if you can even do it. Take a moment to think about what your values are.

These beliefs can sound like reality. They can sound like reality because they represent our past experiences. It must be valid because that is how it has always been. Right?

What is a belief?

Here is some food for thought ... Values are just ideas that we have thought for a long time. We think them so much that our brain recognizes them as truth and fact. For others, we have been exposed to these particular thoughts from a very early age and have kept these views from childhood.

It is important to take these values out and have a look at them. Just like a good closet cleanout, you can find certain values that are very helpful and make you feel amazing. Others will be poor fits and hold you back in your weight loss efforts. Then there will be the sneaky ones. The ones that can sound so factual that you have never contemplated a different way of thinking. Or they're just going to be under the surface, and they're going to feel difficult to get a hold of to look at them.

The good news is that the more you examine your convictions, the easier it becomes to pluck out the tricky ones and look at them.

Why bother with shifting beliefs?

Beliefs become self-fulfilling prophecies. What you spend time thinking about is what you're going to see in life.

So if you have a belief that you can't lose weight, guess what ... You are most likely going to have a hard time losing weight! You won't be able to resist that food if you believe you can't resist XYZ food.

So often, our beliefs are negative and limiting when it comes to weight. They're holding us back. They are tripping us up. Because of what we think, we make the path harder and longer.

You've got the power!

We have the ability, as humans, to choose our thoughts. Here's great news! Because, but some beliefs hold us back, many beliefs can fire you up and propel you forward directly to your aims no matter what gets in your way.

All it takes is to find the right thought and to choose to think it over and over again intentionally.

These fresh thoughts may feel uncomfortable and hard to believe at first. Even when you're not sure you believe them, it's necessary to continue practicing them. Our brains believe over and over what they are told. If you think the same thought over and over purposefully, your brain will start to believe it.

And the reality is, your brain is already doing this. It is thinking thoughts already and believing them as fact. The distinction is that you get to be in the seat of the driver and choose what those thoughts are.

The next steps to take

So sit down and ask yourself what you'd like to believe in your journey towards weight loss. Do you want to believe that it's going to be easy? Or that no matter what gets in your way, you'll remain focused on it? Perhaps, for the last time, you want to believe that you're finding this out.

Choose a conviction that feels secure and gives you optimistic and supportive emotions. Then repeatedly try it to see how much you can amaze yourself!

Most people have heard of The Influence of Belief and restricting beliefs. Still, this idea has been taken up by the scientific community and brought us the amazing reality that the beliefs we hold impact every cell in our body, every relationship we have our everyday actions.

Two Minds of Yours

We've got two minds: conscious and subconscious.

Conscious ones:

- It consists only of the thoughts you intentionally choose to think about.
- It only contributes to 5% of our daily behavior.

Unconscious

- As a man thinks in his heart, so is he," Prov 23:7, "Your subconscious is your true heart and identity.
- Controls how life is perceived, how we respond to circumstances, what we think about ourselves, and what we can achieve.
- Based on every thought, action, emotion, and experience we have ever had in life, it is programmed.
- Your subconscious is what runs 95% of the time.
- When you are not conscientiously thought (when your mind wanders, when you respond to circumstances without thought, even when you are driving, even you know you have zoned out), your subconscious is what is running and driving you on autopilot.

Your Reality

- Perception is reality. We are all perceiving this life entirely differently right now, depending on the filter of our specific subconscious.

- Whatever the reality is, is the reality of the subconscious. You do not become what you think, you be what you believe, and all convictions are contained in the subconscious.
- We want what is in our unconscious to be in line with the person we would like to be- most of the time, it is not.

THE POWER OF BELIEVE

An impressive study exploring the influence of faith and the mind was carried out. This study took 84 hotel attendants with cleaning duties and told half of them that their daily work fulfilled the Surgeon General's guidelines for an active lifestyle as exercise. They just said nothing to the other half.

" As a result, compared with the control group, they showed a decline in weight, blood pressure, body fat, waist-to-hip ratio, and body mass index. These findings support the theory that, through the placebo effect, exercise affects health in part or in full.

That's unbelievable! Our thoughts about food and exercise will alter our bodies physically.

Common Restricting Belief

- I need to prove my worth
- Since I will fail, I can not fulfill my dreams.
- Lack (I have insufficient time, resources, energy)
- I'm not enough (good, educated, slim, young, smart, rich enough).
- I have to make people happy so that I will not be rejected.
- I can't be content before he/she improves.
- I have to gain the approval of other people to feel good about myself.
- I ought to be farther along than I am.
- Whatever I'm doing, I should be doing something else.

You might not even know you have any of these convictions, but if you become conscious that you may, then you may change them. Do any of these resonate with you?

Take Down

1. We do not get what we want; we get what we believe. We may have limiting principles holding us back in some aspects of our life.

2. Fear can kill the most powerful protocol, and that faith can recover with no protocol at all- whatever you really believe defines your outcome: your body, health, performance, and relationships.

What are your beliefs?

You could have a ' program or belief '(way of thinking, or bad habit) that has become something your do automatically and pushes you each day and maybe keeping you back in some areas of your life.

- Where is one place you feel stuck in?
- What is one attitude you keep coming back to?
- What region of life do you view negatively?
- What bad habit should you not stop?
- What health problem are you dealing with?

The source of it is in your subconscious.

You may have personality characteristics or mindsets that have become automatic for you—seeing failure? Negativity? Negativeness? Egotistic? About anxiety? A lack of trust? When we understand that these are all only learned and memorized thoughts, the great news is, they can all be changed!

- What is one oppressive confidence that you want to crack through?

PEELING THE ONION TO WEIGHT LOSS

The numbers look bleak for those of us looking to shed our excess baggage forever.

More than 80 percent of individuals who successfully lose weight gain it back (and more) in just two years, according to a UCLA study of 31 long-term diet studies.

So, why is the law rather than the exception, the yoyo diet? Why are so many of us trapped on the merry-go-round weight loss "gain-lose-gain"?

When you remove an onion all the way, layer after layer, what is left? The Center.

Similarly, what is at the root after eliminating all of the factors that we human beings put on weight (including poor diet, low motivation, and lack of exercise)? Mind. Mind.

Here, we're going to delve into why our mind is the most important part of weight loss, and why meditation is the greatest instrument in the world for shedding pounds ... Everlasting.

With "Suboptimal" options, programming our mind

Any svelte body target we set must click with our subconscious mind as the storage vault for our experiences, feelings, and values. Otherwise, our efforts will be for nothing.

The problem is, after years and years of, let's say,' suboptimal' choices, many of us have conditioned our minds.

Every decision we make digs our paths that much deeper, from raiding the fridge at midnight to snacking on fast food between meals to loading up when we feel down.

Although we may be able to cut carbs and adopt P90x to drop a fast ten pounds, we must ensure that the intensity and consistency of our thoughts are at the highest level if we want to be permanently lean and mean.

What is the right way to do this? Through meditation.

Meditation Unleashes Our Mind Power Unconscious

Sometimes, the human mind is likened to an iceberg.

Since our deeply ingrained habitual, compulsive, and addictive thoughts eventually play out in our conscious mind "over the surface," we need to dive deep beneath the surface to recognize and correct the issue.

In essence, since meditation is the very act of interfacing with our deepest layers of mind, the millennia-old activity is the ideal instrument for the job.

The weight loss game changes as we gain understanding and eventual control of our subconscious mind through meditation.

By regularly tapping into our inner "Indiana Jones treasure trove," we repave any "feed me now ... or else!" belt-stretching thinking ruts that we might have dug into over the years.

With our self-destructive "chocolate cake is love" mind clear ... make sure every cubic inch of your belly is full of toxic desires of love, achieving our ideal body shifts from wishful thinking to reality.

For those of us trying to tighten up the old waistline, what does this mean?

No more appetite for fast food, no more polishing off a Ben & Jerry's tub to feel "full," no more devouring a whole Doritos bag because you can't "help" literally, old habits are easy to break with meditation.

Knowing the mind on a more profound level

Meditation gets to the nitty-gritty of why we emotionally turn to food by interfacing with our mind at the deepest level:

"Am I eating because today my boss chewed me out? Did my dinner time decision cloud the annoyance of being stuck in traffic for an hour? Am I using calories to smother my loneliness? Am I stuffing myself because I have nothing else to look forward to?"

This greater understanding helps us to understand when our food cravings are the product of "emotional hijacking" and when (as nature intended) our cells genuinely need nutrition.

Meditation filters out the shadowy motives why we unintentionally numb ourselves with food by throwing light on the boogeyman hidden under the bed of our conscious mind.

How Our "Inner Fat Boy" Disciplines Meditation

The relation to our brain runs deep when it comes to weight loss. Some overweight adults face challenges that also stem from childhood.

"Since kindergarten, I've been fat, and who I am ..."

While a bit of a harsh word, even decades down the road, our "inner fat kid's" voice may have us dreaming of Snickers, Butterfinger, and Reese's Bits (or the adult equivalent).

Fortunately, meditation shines a light on our mind's deepest, darkest depths, helping us to purge any darkness that can hold us back.

In other words, our inner fat kid is being sent off to boot camp through meditation, bringing him through the wringer, and building him back into a highly disciplined fighter.

Meditation could be the only possible long-term cure for people trying to overcome their weight loss demons.

"Thinking Diets" out of the water Blow "Food Diets."

Neuroscientists claim that the human mind considers 70,000 + thoughts every day. It's only one thinking every two seconds to take out our trusty TI-85 graphing calculator!

And this is for average folks only. Some of us who are at war with the scale also has a far more busy mind.

"I hate my body ... What does it matter if I eat the whole package, I'm fat anyway, I'm fat anyway ... What a lousy day at work, finishing off this angel food cake will make me forget my worries ... I'm doomed to be chubby, I've always been that way and will always ... It's impossible to lose weight, I'm hopeless ..."

Meditation infuses our 'vitamin deficient' mind with exactly what it needs to make healthier lifestyle decisions by placing us on a highly nutritious 'thinking diet.'

In addition to making us much more conscious of what we put in our bodies, the strong relaxation and relaxing of the so-called "monkey mind" through meditation removes two of the main causes, so many of us overeat in the first place: anxiety and depression.

Meditation opens up an entirely new range of advantages, above and beyond being a master of the bathroom scale, with inspiration, great sleep, performance, less anxiety, less depression, and supercharged wellbeing only at the beginning.

AMAZING TIPS & TRICKS FOR SELF-HYPNOSIS TO CALM WORKING PROFESSIONALS

The origin of Self-Hypnosis or Auto-Hypnosis, a type of self-induced hypnosis as it is widely called, can be traced back to 1841 when the word "hypnotism" was first coined. This method of hypnosis is now commonly used and recommended to provide respite from their routine work and life issues to busy professionals.

Although listening to music or a short walk have become the most common ways of self-relaxation for professionals, self-hypnosis is rapidly gaining popularity due to its undisputed and rapid impact on the body and mind of professionals. Most importantly, anytime and anywhere, self-hypnosis can be done so that you do not need a particular time or place to allow your body to relax.

Here are only a few basic methods for self-relaxation that professionals may follow:

Waterfall Technique-This good self-hypnosis approach will relieve you of stress in minutes. All you need to do is take a deep breath and simply imagine a steady stream of hot/cold water flowing either behind or in front of you, containing healing energies. First, visualize and feel yourself walking through this stunning waterfall and the water's calming energies flowing right to your toes through your palms, shoulders, and every other part of your body.

Breathing technique Deep breathing is one of the key points of any form of hypnosis technique. When you imagine the fresh air filling every nook and corner of your lungs, hands, toes, and other distant parts of your body, a simple way is to begin breathing softly, accompanied by deep breathing. Try to imagine the fresh air breeze traveling through your body over the sore spots, and you can feel your body relaxed and revitalized immediately.

Mini Power Nap Technique This approach is particularly useful and recommended for continually feeling lethargic and exhausted at work. For a few minutes, the procedure allows you to sit or lie down, followed by a deep breath when attempting to locate your body's pain points. If you have understood the points, recommend that your body release the stresses and fill the room with fresh energy flow. When your body starts to relax while reminding yourself to feel revitalized when you wake up after the power nap, get ready for a charged-up hypnosis power nap.

So, if you're a workaholic and can sense your body wanting quick relaxation, try one of these methods of self-hypnosis and sense the magic for yourself!!

SEVEN CONSTRUCTIVE WAYS TO REWIRE YOUR SELF FOR RESILIENCE

When you face difficulties in your life, do you feel ready to handle it or get exhausted and trapped in the struggle, grief, or even the unfairness of your situation? If you are facing an injury, career transition, divorce, family hardship, or any other significant problem, there are strategies you can use to create confidence and rewire your brain for resilience.

1. Embrace the strength or weakness

" Vulnerability is not weakness. And the myth is deeply dangerous, " says insecurity and bravery specialist, Brene Brown. When I became a mum for the first time last year, I learned that being genuine and vulnerable was key to building resilience.

In the early days and our little guy was not sleeping well, unnerved, and crying all night, I quickly became overwhelmed. All I needed to do was sleep, have a break, and, at moments, go back to my old life with all its independence.

In those particularly difficult days, I let myself experience what I was feeling. Some days it meant sitting on the bathroom floor and having a good cry; other days, it was having a frank talk with my husband or mum about how hard I was finding it. It most assurances meant asking for and welcoming support.

At first, I felt bad for feeling and thinking this way. I wondered if I was a " bad parent" for not enjoying every minute of motherhood. To be vulnerable, it took courage and let my guard down. "Once I got over the guilt, however, I discovered that letting myself" unravel "released built-up emotions and created space in my mind to reconnect with my inner strength and think," OK, Jess, get up and keep going, you can do this!

Your brain has switched gears, and your limbic system, the emotional engine of your brain, has taken over while you are in a highly dynamic condition. This makes it more difficult to think clearly and to stay on top of the problems and challenges. You will relieve some of the emotions you feel by recognizing and expressing your feelings and thoughts. This helps to relax the nervous system and "dials down" the reaction to fight or flight.

Your pre-frontal cortex, the logical thinking part of your brain, will step in when the emotional part of your brain is no longer in overdrive. Your pre-frontal cortex will help you more clearly see your condition and encourage you to feel more positive about your ability to cope with your challenges and setbacks and rise above them.

To get through a difficult time you are facing, do you need to ask for help and support? Who should you have an honest conversation with to clear out some room in your mind?

2. Choose your concentration

It can be frustrating when things in life do not go to plan. Your brain immediately focuses your mind on your issues when your stress response is activated. Neuroscientist Dr. Rick Hanson claims that as part of the coping system, the brain is like Velcro for unpleasant experiences and is, in reality, hard-wired to bind to negative experiences.

This narrowing of your attention on your issues restricts your ability to react to the problems in your life in a resilient way and causes your brain to continue to see only what does not work. Have you ever found that something goes wrong when you're having a 'bad day'? The traffic is sluggish these days, there are no parking areas at work, and the stores are closed when you get there ... the list goes on.

You are not aware of the positive things that are happening and what you have in your life to be thankful for, whereas your brain focuses on the issues around you. Your understanding and interpretation of life are generated by what you concentrate on. "Consider these questions to "unstick" your brain from dwelling on your issues: "What is going well in my life? And "What is the flip-side of this challenge or situation?"

3. Become consciously grateful. Gratitude keeps your brain from concentrating on what you have lost and what has changed and turns your mind on what you still have and what you should be grateful for.

It is an important part of resilience to see what is still possible despite the challenges. Becoming consciously grateful helped me restore my life in my twenties when I was diagnosed with a chronic illness.

Initially, when I became sick, I was all consumed by what I had lost, but then I could see that I still had the potential to contribute by writing from my bed, even though I could no longer work a regular 9-5 job or do most daily stuff. You train your brain to pay attention to the good around you as you consciously go searching for things for which to be grateful.

In so doing, you get a more optimistic view of your life. You will also start feeling better, as gratitude stimulates the reward system in your brain and releases dopamine, one in your feel-good chemicals. It is as easy to be consciously thankful as taking a moment each day to think about at least three unique items for which you are grateful.

They can be as large as "I'm grateful for my family's help," or as tiny as "I'm grateful that today I had time to sit down and have a hot cup of coffee." You can begin to appreciate even the smallest items that have given you pleasure during the day when you become deliberately grateful.

You may also find that in time you become thankful for the hardship itself. Resilience specialist, keynote speaker, and quadriplegic Stacey Copas say in her book, How To Be Resilient, " Most people find it hard to believe that growing up as a quadriplegic and having to use a wheelchair for the rest of my life is a good thing ... but I am genuinely happy about it. I have done things in my life that I can claim in confidence I would never have done. "

Are you focused on the negatives or the positives of your life? Looking back on your life, are you thankful for any adversities you faced? What did they tell you?

4. Reframe the challenge

According to psychologist Angela Duckworth in her novel, Grit, the feeling that you have some influence over your life is key to hope, determination, and resilience. When it comes to overcoming challenges, you may not alter what has happened to you, but you can choose how you view and react to the situation.

Dr. John Arden, in his novel, Re-Wire Your Brain, says, " The emotional tone and viewpoint with which you define each experience will potentially rewire your brain. The more you explain your ongoing experience in a specific way, the stronger the neural circuits that reflect those thoughts become. Your narratives can be positive or negative. "What you tell yourself as you face obstacles can decide how much you come back. I found this to be particularly true after giving birth to my son, as the birth didn't go smoothly.

I was induced and ended up having an emergency cesarean at 38 weeks. After 12 hours of intense yet unsuccessful labor, the cesarean occurred, an epidural that did not work and increasing fears for my son. I was more than relieved to see our beautiful boy and know that he was safe and healthy, but it was an experience that left my mind with fear.

I had gone expecting and waiting for normal childbirth, and I was disappointed that it was a positive birth experience not to get what I felt. I realized I needed to reframe the narrative I had chosen to find peace and healing around this encounter.

"To change my perspective, I asked myself," What is the positive experience of birth? I learned something powerful by turning my mind away from all that went wrong and all my frustrated expectations: I had experienced an extremely positive birth experience because my son was born alive and safe, and I was extremely thankful for that.

Stepping back and asking yourself multiple questions will give you a new viewpoint that is more helpful. Is there a scenario that you have framed that you might reframe negatively? What story about this situation do you say yourself? What does this cost you emotionally? Is there a more constructive way for this situation to be viewed?

5. Switch to a mentality of solution

"Resilience consists of preserving the expectation that things will ultimately change in the face of hardship while doing what it takes to make certain things happen," Arden says. In your life, taking action, no matter how small, generates momentum and trust and gives you back power.

Weighing back on what has happened will make it impossible to concentrate on finding a solution to the issue at hand. Think of the next action explicitly, not a series of actions down the road or the series of actions that have gone before,' Copas says.

Reactivate your pre-frontal cortex to cultivate a solution-focused mentality by asking yourself a series of questions that motivate more critical thinking, concentrating on solutions, and moving forward. To create resilience, ask yourself:

- What power do I still have?
- What help do I have around me that I can make better use of?
- What other assets do I have that would support me?
- What is one tiny thing that I can do to shift my life in a better direction right now?

6. Visualize a positive future

You may have noticed that your heart begins to race when you imagine something stressful, your stomach may feel queasy, and your palms may feel sweaty. It is only by the images you play through your mind that your fight-or-flight response can be activated. What you imagine greatly affects your brain. Studies demonstrate that when you imagine something and do it, the same neural pathways light up.

Positive visualization allows you to deliberately replace with best-case scenarios any worst-case scenarios running through your mind that will allow you to feel confident and optimistic. For instance, you could visualize yourself confidently attending interviews, answering questions with ease, and landing your dream job if you were facing a career change, instead of imagining being out of work for months.

Neuroscientist Dr. Sarah McKay explains that you need to imagine yourself in the scenario to create a powerful visualization, not imagine yourself from the perspective of an outsider. She also states that you need to practice your scenario frequently to get the most out of positive visualization. You can write out your best-case scenario and read it back to yourself to practice your visualizations, or record yourself saying it on your phone and listen to it while commuting or before going to bed.

Are you running through your mind a worst-case scenario that makes you anxious? What would it look like in your best-case scenario? When could you practice throughout your day to visualize this scenario?

7. Safeguard your energy

Responding to life, resiliently takes energy. Be aware of what helps you feel relaxed, happy, confident, and supported, and make time for those experiences to keep your brain and body energized.

Remain in the moment. There are times when the big picture will undermine your resilience, and you will be drained of the energy and trust you need to keep going. You can help your brain stay calm and in control by focusing on each day as it comes (or even every hour) and keep away from overwhelming.

Ten Ways to Remain Energized

- Do not compare your trip to others.
- Accept and ask for assistance and support
- Prioritizing sleep and rest
- Moving your body routinely
- Build healthy limits and say no when you need to
- Eat a wholesome and balanced diet
- Spend 5-10 minutes a day concentrating on breathing or meditation.
- Connecting with loved ones
- Changing your setting and spending time in nature
- Joke as much as possible

It's never easy to go through challenging times, but when you can take care of how your brain sparks and wires, you can deal with the obstacles in your life effectively and rewire your brain for greater strength and motivation and a much brighter future

Chapter 7: 9 SIMPLE WAYS TO QUICKLY BOOST YOUR SELF-ESTEEM

Your level of self-esteem will determine how you feel about yourself and what you believe you can do. With these ten easy tips, find out how to build your self-esteem.

High self-esteem, individuals believe in themselves and their skills. Low self-esteem can, on the other hand, make us feel doubtful and critical of ourselves and our abilities.

Also, low self-esteem can make you blame yourself for things beyond your control and prevent meaningful relationships from developing.

What does self-esteem mean?

First, understanding the term esteem, which means admiring, approving, like, appreciating, or holding in high regard, is important.

Self-esteem, therefore, refers to the degree of self-worth, self-love, self-approval, self-confidence, or self-respect you have.

Self-esteem, in other words, means you can positively view yourself.

What's more, it means that, regardless of your shortcomings or errors, you are still capable of loving yourself. Having said that, based on your day-to-day experiences, how you feel and think about yourself can differ.

Unfortunately, low self-esteem is a self-fulfilling prophecy. The less motivation you have to do what it takes to build your self-esteem, the worse you feel about who you are and what you do.

It's easy to spiral from there into a cycle of negative and circular thinking, keeping you mired in harmful beliefs—and erroneous ones.

How can you stop this vicious cycle and start going in a more productive direction for yourself?

It's a phase, and it won't happen overnight, but there are things you can do to get it started and keep it going. Here are 20 effective ways to boost your self-esteem quickly to start feeling more positive.

1. Learn a new ability.

When you become professional at something that correlates with your abilities and interests, you improve your sense of competency.

2. List your achievements.

Dream of all the things you've done and written them down. Create a list of everything you've done that you feel proud of, everything you've done well. Check your list when you need a reminder of your desire to get stuff done and do them well.

3. Do something imaginative.

Creative activities are a perfect way to bring the rhythm back into your life. Creativity activates the brain, but the more you use it, the greater the benefits. Pull out your old guitar, write a story or essay, take a dance class, or sign up for a community theater production. When you add the obstacle of trying something new, it inspires you even more.

4. Get specific on your principles.

Determine what your beliefs are and evaluate your life to see if you're not living in harmony with what you believe. Then make the necessary adjustments. The more you know what you stand for, the more confident you will be.

5. Challenge the restricting values.

When you find yourself thinking negatively about yourself, stop, and question yourself. Don't let yourself be constrained by erroneous beliefs.

6. Stand at the edge of your comfort zone.

Stretch yourself and step to the edge of your comfort zone. Get uncomfortable — try something new, meet different people, or handle a situation unusually. Esteem starts at the edge of your comfort zone.

7. Somebody support.

To support others, use your strengths, abilities, and skills. Offer direct assistance to someone, share helpful tools, or teach what they want to learn to someone. As a present to someone, give anything you do well.

8. Heal your past.

Unresolved problems and drama will keep you stuck in low self-esteem. Seek the guidance of a professional counselor to help you heal the past so you can step into the future in a secure and self-assured way.

9. Stop thinking about what others think.

When you worry about what people will think about you, you never feel free to be yourself. Make a firm commitment to stop thinking about what other people think — begin making decisions based on what you want, not what you think others want from you.

10. Learn something inspiring.

A perfect way to achieve more self-esteem is to read something that lifts you and makes you feel good about yourself.

11. Reclaim your honor.

Define what honesty means for you, and ensure that you're living in compliance with that understanding. If your life isn't consistent with your character, it will exhaust you and leave you feeling bad about yourself.

12. Let go of negative people.

If there are people who are negative in your life — who have nothing good to say or who are putting you down or taking advantage of you — do the smart thing and let them go. The best way to find self-esteem is to surround yourself with optimistic, compassionate individuals who respect and appreciate you.

13. In the sand, draw a line.

Building personal limits is the perfect way to discover your self-esteem. Know what your limits are, and when people cross them, how you want to react. Don't allow others to dominate you, exploit you, or take advantage of you. To be assured is the protection of strong limits.

14. Take care of your look.

You feel your best when you look your best. Dress like someone who has faith and in how you look, let your self-assurance show through.

15. Welcoming failure as part of growth.

When you've lost, it's a normal answer to be tough on yourself. But if you can change your thinking to realize that failure is a chance to learn, it plays a vital role in learning and development; it can enable you to retain perspective. Bear in mind that failure also means you are making an effort.

16. Remain a student.

As a lifelong learner, think about yourself. Approach anything you do with the mindset of a student — what Shoshin or "beginner's mind" is called by Zen Buddhists — open, ready, impartial, and willing to learn.

17. Face the anxiety.

Enable yourself to feel frightened, but anyway, keep ongoing.

In the dance between your deepest desires and your greatest fears, self-esteem is always sought.

18. Become an advisor.

For anyone who needs your help, your leadership, and your encouragement, be there. Their love and gratitude—and seeing them progress with your help—will contribute to your self-esteem and self-respect.

19. Define achievement.

Clarify what success means to you in terms of your confidence and what it means. You'll have to find the self-esteem inside yourself to just do it if you want to do something.

Chapter 8: 30 KNOWN WAYS THAT WEIGHT LOSS WILL CHANGE YOUR LIFE

While we can feel like our lives are pretty boring, the fact is that people are ever-evolving; we are all experiencing various things that change who we are and change our everyday lives. And while there's no denying that things are big deals, like getting married or beginning your dream career, few things are as transformative as weight loss, particularly when it's a large amount. And that's because their weight determines, for many, how they feel about themselves and how others see them. Our body image defines how we connect with others, how positive we feel, and how safe we feel in our everyday lives. When you lose those excess pounds and hit your target size, there are plenty of weight loss benefits that come your way!

So, while you've already trained yourself psychologically for some of the changes associated with slimming down (i.e., buying new pants), there are a variety of weight-loss advantages, as well as some unusual changes, you may never have known that a trimmer figure comes along with it. Read on to explore the benefits of losing the pounds, and check out these ways to lose weight and keep it off to preserve your sexy new body for life while you're at it!

1.Maybe you'll get a raise.

Infuriating but true: After you've slimmed down, your boss may treat you better. According to a study in Health Economics, obese individuals, especially women, make around 2.5 percent less than their normal-weight co-workers. Although that may not sound too spectacular, that's the difference between making $60,000 and $61,500 a year. That's enough spare cash to buy a fancy designer bag or go on a holiday!

Dropping down to a healthier weight can also up the chances of landing a promotion, according to a recent University of Surrey and University of Oxford study. The psychologists behind the study discovered that weight and perceived beauty both play a major part in whether or not anyone can secure their dream work or score a promotion. They have essentially found that the heavier the person, the lower their chances. It gets worse: your chances of career advancement are much smaller than your male counterparts if you're an overweight woman.

2.You can say so long. For seasonal allergies,

Your weight may have been to blame if your eyes used to itch every spring until the flowers began to bloom. Being overweight, exacerbating asthma and allergy symptoms can strain the adrenal glands and respiratory system. You might be able to ditch your inhaler and cut down on the seasonal pill-popping now that you're trimmer, but don't do so without talking to your M.D. Uh, first! After you've dropped the meds, still sniffling? Make this to eat, not that! Your Seasonal Bible to Cure Spring Allergies.

3.The food is going to taste better.

Get this: Your dinner can taste even better after losing weight. Overweight individuals have less openness to taste than their slimmer peers, according to a report by Stanford University. This may be because taste buds become dulled from overuse, the experts behind the study claim.

Eat it! Tip Tip

Try nutritious foods that you've never liked before. They can become new favorites in your trimmer frame, which will help you sustain your weight loss in the long run.

4.You may have the opportunity to throw your meds.

You already know that problems like heart disease and diabetes can be avoided by achieving a healthier weight, but did you know that losing weight can also help relieve the effects of your current conditions? That means you can be able to take your current drugs at reduced doses or avoid taking those medicines entirely. (Which saves lots of cash for you!) Check-in with your M.D. And see what sorts of improvements he or she feels the slimmer you might benefit from.

5.It'll boost your sex drive.

Nope, it's not about your talent. You are aroused more quickly as your BMI dips, and it's all thanks to increasing levels of testosterone. Heavier men had T-levels comparable to gents nearly a full decade older in one Journal of Clinical Endocrinology & Metabolism research. In the nude, you may even feel less self-conscious, which can also increase your urge to get it on.

6.And you're just going to love sex more.

Before you lose weight if you thought sex was nice, wait until you get into it in your new, leaner body! In a Duke University Medical Center study of 1,210 individuals of different weights, obese individuals were 25 times more likely than their leaner peers to report disappointment with their time between the sheets. The best of all news? In the study, sexual pleasure was shown to skyrocket by a mere 10% loss of body weight. So, even though you're always not quite where you want to be with your physique, you can always reap in the bedroom the rewards. And be sure to nosh on a couple of these foods for better sex, to make your romp even warmer!

7.It'll seem better for your work.

Slimmer body, more intelligent brain? Probably. According to a study published in the journal Frontiers in Nutrition, heavier men have worse cognitive abilities than trimmer men.

8.The sofa is going to look less appealing.

Before you lost weight, those extra LBs hurt your knees and physically weighed you down. So it isn't shocking that you were exhausted and craving couch time on the reg. Your knees will hopefully feel less achy now,that you've lost the weight, though, and your energy levels will increase, making your oh-so-squishy couch look less enticing.

9.There might be changed in your goals.

The blogger behind Hungry Safe Happy, Dannii Martin, lost a whopping 98 pounds in 18 months after her doc told her that she had developed heart problems. She writes in a blog entitled "Losing Weight Did Change Me-I Am Not The Same Person," "My priorities have changed. Going out and drinking used to revolve around my life, and my life is much more balanced now. [My priorities now] include tasks, good food (occasionally junk, mostly healthy), spending time with the people I love, exercising, and being happy in general. Of course, there are still so many."

10.You'll sleep better.

They may seem entirely unrelated, but there is a curious connection between snoring, sleep, and weight loss. With a weight loss of as little as five percent, sleep apnea and snoring, often caused by excess weight around the neck, can disappear. So, you'll sleep better once you've lost some weight, which will help drive your weight loss gains even more! Check out these things to do before bed to lose weight to make the most of your nighttime slumber.

11.Maybe, you're more relaxed.

Before losing an amazing 150-pounds, Fred Lechuga, who pens the Fat 2 Fit Fred blog, used to have terrible road rage. But he said he's cool as a cucumber since he's been losing weight. In his bookkeeping weight It Off: Life After Losing 100 Pounds, he writes: "When I was overweight, and behind the wheel, when I went to and from work, my middle finger was out the window quite a bit. (I know, I know, stupid.) Nowadays, my attitude is more like," Whatever dude, cut me off, I don't care.

12.Maybe your memory will improve.

If it has been a challenge for you most of your life to recall the names of people, the extra weight you carried around may have been to blame. In one study, after losing weight, women performed better on memory tests than they did before falling pounds. About why? Brain scans found that after women lost weight, during memory retrieval, there was more activity when they were forming memories and less activity, indicating that carrying extra pounds around could make it more difficult for the brain to function effectively. Be sure to steer clear of these high-fat foods that damage your brain to ensure that you can remember crucial information late in life.

13.It'll plummet your tolerance.

She got over 3,257 comments when Reddit user Digbybare asked fellow "formerly obese Redditors" to share their "most surprising/unexpected improvement since losing weight"! And for some perspective, you can bet we dug through a decent share of them! MattressCrane writes in response to the query: "I've been down about 50 pounds since this October, and I find that I get considerably intoxicated from unexpectedly small amounts of alcohol whenever I drink. No more nine beers to get buzzed for me. I suppose, just another advantage." Fewer calories and fewer dollars wasted, certainly a win!

14.You will observe all of the seasons.

Another common theme among weight loss editors? Being very cold all the time, like. Some of them also said that for the first time in years since their weight loss, they wanted to invest in a nice winter coat! And it makes sense; if you lose as little as 10% of your body weight, the levels of thyroid hormones will drop, which can make you feel cold more often than not, says Judith Korner, director of the Columbia University Medical Center's Weight Management Center. For the colder months, invest in a coat and keep those sweaters and hoodies on hand around the clock, people!

15. Maybe you'll clash more with your partner.

We have already told you that losing weight will make your sex life better, so that must mean that being a skinny Minnie will also boost your romantic relationships, right? Not fully. Instead, relationship specialists advise that after losing the pounds, the partner might feel threatened. They may worry that more people will provide you with romantic attention, or they may feel dissatisfied with your new healthier lifestyle, particularly if they know that they can also make changes to improve their health. The main thing is that you don't let tension dissuade you from holding your trimmer figure with your partner. It can help to prepare you emotionally and be able to talk with your partner about it by simply being conscious that this will happen.

16.Amusement parks would be more enjoyable.

One of the most surprising and funny responses we came across on the Reddit forum came from user Justcallmezach, who had recently lost a considerable amount of weight: "The first time I jumped into a go-kart and flew around the track, I was freaking shocked. I thought the karts had been upgraded; then, I just realized they were [going much faster] when they were hauling 135 [fewer] pounds."

17.Your cancer risk would be lower.

While most people know that factors can raise their cancer risk, such as smoking and having too much sun, few individuals understand that obesity is also linked to cancer. (It is to blame for disease-causing inflammation caused by obesity.) That is bad news. The good news is that, according to a Cancer Research study of postmenopausal women, levels of inflammation can be decreased by losing just five percent of your body weight. And there were similar findings in a study on morbidly obese men who underwent bariatric surgery. It sounds like a cause for us to celebrate with one of these tasty smoothies for weight loss!

18.You're going to become a gym rat.

It's not unusual for exercises to induce a burning sensation in your lungs when you're carrying extra pounds around. It's also not rare for the joints to be in a lot of discomforts. For this reason, exercise will begin to feel more like fun and less like a chore until the weight begins to peel off. Plus, what they're saying is true: the feel-good endorphins that enter the body after a killer Zumba class are very addictive. Not to mention, progression is addictive, too! You'll want to keep coming back for more as you continue to lose belly fat and gain muscle.

19.You're not going to be as hungry.

While some dieters report feeling hungrier after slimming down, Fatsecret user Deana Garcia writes on the message board that she "eats much less" after losing 25 pounds and doesn't "feel hungry all the time" as she used to do. If we had to guess, it's probably because she's consuming nutritious foods filled with nutrients such as protein and fiber. It improves satiety. If you follow a similar slim-down method, while eating less and keeping your trimmer body, you should expect to keep your appetite under wraps.

20. You'll have more money to spend.

According to a Health Affairs survey, those who clock in at a safe weight spend 42 percent less money on medical bills and health costs than their overweight counterparts. And not only a few Benjamins are being saved; these slim minnies spend $1,429 fewer dollars a year than their heavier counterparts do. More money is yet another excuse to get pumped about a leaner body in your pocket.

21.It can improve your hair and skin.

Reddit user Oppiken said that after losing weight, his skin cleared up, and his hair started looking cleaner and less limp. Since many nutrients found in healthy foods have beautifying advantages, it is fair to say that his weight loss diet is likely to thank him for his enhanced appearance. Would you like to lose weight and also boost your complexion? Connect these superior skin health foods to your weekly lineup.

22.Who your true friends are, you find out.

There's no denying it: so do the relationships as the body shifts. Most of your friends would be pleased with you, but a few will be jealous and resentful, particularly if your relationship is based on a shared understanding of what it is like to be overweight. If it happens to you, ask a friend of yours what's up. Tell them you appreciate their friendship, and ask them if you should talk about why they behaved differently towards you. You will usually work it out if they are open to talking about it.

23.You are going to sweat less.

You wear a weighted vest in a hot room 24/7 when you're overweight, which is no simple feat. (The body is protected by fat and the core temperature increases.) This is why obese people appear to sweat more than their slimmer counterparts. Reddit user somebunnylovesyou said her sweat stains were so bad before losing weight that she would have to get to class 15 minutes early to clean herself with wet towels in the bathroom. She is excited to say after dropping the pounds that she no longer gets all sweaty and "no longer worries about kissing individuals."

24.Maybe people are nicer to you.

Although it's not completely appropriate, our culture emphasizes being slim, which is why overweight people are discriminated against or unfairly handled. In reality, it is such a concern that obesity researchers will also use something called a Fat Phobia Scale, a weight bias determination questionnaire, to ensure that their study findings are not affected. That said, after you've lost weight, it could feel like you're traveling through an alternate universe every day. People who have snubbed you once may welcome you with a smile, and people may even do little things to give you a hand or hold doors for you, including going out of their way. "Now I've lost 120 pounds, and people treat me a lot differently.

25.Your energy is going to skyrocket.

You may have found that you had much more stamina after falling those pounds. This isn't about the more healthy food that you eat, either. Simply put, the body uses less energy when you're lugging around less weight to keep you alive. It has also been shown that slimming down increases the use of oxygen, so you probably won't get as windy walking up the stairs or looking after your little ones.

26.For help, people will come to you.

It makes sense: people would want to come to you for help when they see that you've lost pounds! Be proud of the motivation and direction people are searching for you, be transparent and frank about what worked for you, and share the obstacles you had to conquer.

27.You will become more unforgettable.

One thing became painfully apparent after reading through various message boards for individuals who have recently trimmed down: they thought people were noticing them more. One user writes, "When I first lost weight, guys paid me much more respect ... After becoming kind of invisible because of my weight, I found it difficult to get used to it." Another user adds, "I lost 100 pounds. The most shocking thing to me was that I'm no longer mistaken for anyone else. When you're 300 + pounds, the overweight is recognized by all people. [Many people think] all fat people look the same."

28 .You could become more judgmental.

[Since losing weight,] on the sidewalks, I blast by people and get irritated with overweight people now, "Reddit user R3solv writes." Whenever I see a person who is overweight, I want to tell them that there is a better way! But I've got to keep my mouth shut because that would just be disrespectful, you know. This raccoon agrees: "That, too, happened to me!" I suddenly realized that I was secretly criticizing obese people, especially those with carts full of garbage at the grocery store. I don't understand this. Shouldn't I, as an ex-fat guy, really be more understanding? If you feel judgmental, take a step back and refocus on your actions, not someone else's.

29.Maybe you don't know like you look now.

Countless heavy individuals assume that after losing weight, their body morale will get an instant boost, but for many, that's not how the story goes. "It took me a while to be able to feel the way I looked after losing weight, and I'm still not quite there," admits Fatsecret message board user anna Sankar. I was 167 pounds and a size 12 two years ago. Now I'm 120 pounds, and I'm wearing a size 2 or 4, but I still feel like I should wear an eight or a 10! "She goes on to say that your exterior and interior have a" massive emotional link. "She says," It takes time for you to recognize your new body. No matter how many people tell you how thin you look, before you can see it for yours.

30. A longer life, you'll live.

A slimmer you = a longer lifespan. Maybe you already knew that.

How would your body adjust when you start eating nutritious food?

One day after starting

Throughout the day, you will have fewer food cravings,

eventually feeling in control of your food choices. This encourages you to reach for healthier food, setting yourself up for long-term weight loss and fitness success instead of the less nutritious you might have preferred before.

You can see the hunger has stabilized. You may have noticed that you feel ravenous before 10 a.m. And 3 p.m., but now you're never troubled by the pains of hunger. It makes weight loss feel so much simpler.

You will feel a greater degree of mental attention and clarification. As you begin to find that you can think more clearly, any signs of brain fog or poor concentration should start to clear up.

You'll feel shocked that without gaining weight, you can consume so much food. You may also feel excessively full for the first few days of healthy eating. However, stick with it as the feeling will pass, and you will feel better than you've ever had before.

One week after beginning

Your level of energy is greater than you might have ever experienced before, making it easier to complete everyday tasks and even exercise!). In reality, you will find that you are looking forward to your workout sessions because now you finally have the power to do them.

You may begin to find that your pants feel looser than before. Owing to high sodium intake, the body will shed all the extra water you have stored, along with so many previously refined foods. In the mirror, this even comes with looking leaner. Your weight on the scale will drop anywhere from 2-5 pounds.

You're beginning to find that your food cravings are lessening. Although you might have wanted pizza, burgers, and ice cream earlier, now you're looking forward to the balanced meals you've scheduled.

You'll find that you are beginning to sleep more properly. You fall more quickly asleep and seem to wake up less all night long.

Your body will become ordinary. This, along with looking slimmer, will come with a smaller amount of bloating and discomfort.

Your moods are more stable, you will note. Throughout the day, you have fewer ups and downs and might even start to feel more empowered in your everyday life.

One month after getting started

You'll find that your skin has a new glow. People can start reflecting on how radiant you look and how younger you seem to look.

Depending on what your starting point was, you can now see a steady rate of weight loss (if using a lower calorie approach) to the tune of 1/2 to 2 pounds per week.

Some of the pre-existing health issues (migraines, joint pain, irritable bowel problems, etc.) that you may have endured may begin to clear up. You are finally beginning to feel good for the first time in a long time.

Many people assume that healthy eating is more costly. Still, with this new strategy, you can save money when you add up all the meals you eat out along with the higher-priced convenience products you can purchase (chocolate bars, granola bars, canned goods, etc.).

You will simply reject unhealthy foods that are presented to you. You've come to understand how much better you feel when you don't consume those things for a month and choose to stick to a balanced eating schedule.

Eating right is beginning to become more routine. You'll learn that you naturally want to do it without thinking after doing something for 21 days straight. Making wise decisions can start to feel like second nature.

You will begin to experience enhanced efficiency while you are exercising. In the gym, you can feel better and find that you are healing much quicker when you come out. You feel the 'post-workout glow' that everyone is always talking about, but that you might never have noticed before.

You may find that you are starting to get hungrier. This is due to the stimulation of your metabolism, being used to all the nutritious food that you consume, which comes at regular intervals. Without adding body weight, you can now eat more.

Six months after having begun

If they were on the high side before beginning this strategy, you'd note a drop in your total cholesterol levels.

Your blood pressure can also decrease, reducing your risk of stroke and heart disease.

You should feel visibly thinner as you would have lost 10-30 pounds (if using a reduced-calorie weight loss approach).

Your bones will become stronger, and your chance of stress fractures and breaks will be minimized. Although it's not something you can see, trust that it's going to happen.

Your blood glucose levels will be under much greater control, decreasing the spikes of blood sugar and decreasing the risk factor for diabetes (or the symptoms will be much better controlled if you are still suffering).

A year after starting

You will also reap all of the above-noted benefits as these advantages will remain as long as you continue to eat well.

A bodyweight where you feel safe, heavy, and secure would be at your target weight.

You can find yourself wanting to try new sports/activities/exercises. Finally, you feel like you have reached a point where you believe in physical activity like your body can do.

You're sure you're not going to return to your old lifestyle at this stage—too many positive improvements you've seen to give it all up for certain foods.

You realize how inherently inspired certain individuals appear to be. For you, balanced eating is no longer something you're concentrating on; it's just something you're doing.

You would have learned to indulge wisely by this point, you can treat yourself if you wish, and it won't cause you to fall completely off your plan right away.

You will feel happier and healthier than you have ever experienced before.

Chapter 9: 18 WAYS TO MINIMIZE HUNGER AND APPETITE BASED ON SCIENCE

You usually need to decrease your daily calorie intake to lose weight.

Weight loss diets, sadly, frequently result in increased appetite and extreme hunger.

This can make losing weight and keeping it off incredibly difficult.

Here is a list of 18 ways to minimize excessive hunger and appetite, based on science:

1. Just Eat Enough Protein

Adding more protein to your diet will improve feelings of fullness, make you eat less, and help you lose weight at your next meal.

For example, a report on weight loss compared two calorie-identical breakfasts: one consisting of eggs, the other of bagels.

Over the eight week study period, participants who had the egg breakfast lost 65 percent more weight and 16 percent more body fat.

Moreover, when daily calories are reduced for weight loss, a high intake of protein can help to prevent muscle loss.

To have the benefits, it seems appropriate to make protein between 20-30 percent of the overall calorie intake or 0.45-0.55 g / lb of body weight (1.0-1.2 g / kg).

Having enough protein in your diet, partly by reducing your appetite, will help promote weight loss.

2. Pick Fiber-Rich Foods

A high intake of fiber stretches the stomach, reduces its rate of emptying, and affects the release of hormones for the fullness.

Furthermore, the bowel will ferment fiber. This creates short-chain fatty acids that are thought to help further foster feelings of fullness.

In reality, a recent study reports that adding to your meal fiber-rich beans, peas, chickpeas, and lentils can improve feelings of fullness by 31 percent, compared to comparable meals that are not focused on beans.

Whole grains rich in fiber can also help decrease hunger and keep you feeling whole.

You will reduce your calorie consumption by up to 10 percent by eating an additional 14 grams of fiber per day. It could lead to a loss of up to 4.2 lbs (1.9 kg) over 3.8 months.

More recent studies, however, have found less drastic results. This may have to do with the various fiber forms studied.

More viscous fiber forms such as pectins, beta-glucans, and guar gum tend to be more filling than less dense fiber types.

Moreover, few adverse effects have been associated with high-fiber diets. There are also many other beneficial nutrients in fiber-rich foods, including vitamins, minerals, antioxidants, and helpful plant compounds.

Therefore, long-term wellness can also be promoted by opting for a diet that includes ample fruits, vegetables, beans, nuts, and seeds.

Eating a diet rich in fiber will minimize malnutrition and help you consume fewer calories. It can foster long-term health, as well.

3. Choose Solids Over Liquids

Solid calories and liquid calories can have different effects on your appetite.

One recent analysis showed that people who consumed a liquid snack were 38 percent less likely to compensate by consuming less at the next meal than a solid snack.

Participants served a semi-solid snack in a second study showed less hunger, less urge to eat, and a higher feeling of fullness than those feeding a liquid snack.

Solids require more chewing, which will provide more time to enter the brain for the fullness signal.

Scientists also assume that the additional chewing time helps solids to remain in contact for longer with the taste buds, which may also facilitate feelings of fullness.

Without getting more hungry, eating your calories rather than consuming them will make you eat less.

4. Drink your coffee

Coffee has many health and athletic performance advantages and can also help suppress your appetite.

Research shows that the release of peptide YY (PYY) is stimulated by coffee. In response to feeding, this hormone is produced in the gut and promotes a feeling of fullness.

In deciding how much you are likely to consume, scientists agree that PYY levels play an important role.

Interestingly, decaffeinated coffee, with results that last up to three hours after consumption, will generate the highest reduction in hunger.

However, to pinpoint precisely how this works, further studies are needed.

For up to three hours, drinking coffee, especially decaf, may help reduce hunger.

5. On Water, Fill Up

Before meals, drinking water will help reduce the hunger you experience.

After a meal, it can also increase feelings of fullness and encourage weight loss,

In reality, studies show that people eat 22 percent less than those who do not drink any water when drinking two glasses of water immediately before a meal.

Scientists assume that approximately 17 oz (500 ml) of water is enough to stretch the stomach enough to send fullness signals to the brain.

That said, it is also understood that water empties rapidly from the stomach. It could be better to drink the water as near the meal for this tip to work.

Interestingly, it could be the same way to start your meal with soup.

Researchers found that immediately before a meal, consuming a bowl of soup decreased hunger and lowered the overall intake of calories from the meal by around 100 calories.

Before a meal, consuming low-calorie drinks will help you consume fewer calories without leaving you hungry.

6. Feed Mindfully and Prepare

Your brain knows, under normal circumstances, whether you are hungry or full.

Eating fast or when you're distracted, however, will make it harder for your brain to identify these signals.

Solve this dilemma, a key aspect of mindful eating, by removing distractions and concentrating on the foods in front of you.

Research indicates that it can help people feel more satisfied when eating by practicing mindfulness during meals. This will help sustain the emphasis on quality rather than quantity and reduce the behavior of binge eating.

A relation between hunger, fullness, and what your eyes see also seems to be there.

One experiment gave participants two similar milkshakes. A "620-calorie indulgence" was named one, while a "120-calorie sensible" label was granted to the other.

While both groups ate the same amount of calories, for those who claimed they drank the "indulgent" drink, hunger hormone levels fell more.

Believing that there are more calories in a drink can also cause the brain areas to feel full.

What you see can affect how full you feel, and it can be very helpful to pay attention to what you eat.

It has been shown that mindful eating reduces appetite and increases feelings of fullness. It can also decrease the consumption of calories and help avoid binge eating.

7. Indulge yourself in Dark Chocolate

It is believed that the bitterness of dark chocolate helps to suppress hunger and decrease cravings for sweets.

The stearic acid in dark chocolate can also help slow digestion, further increasing feelings of fullness, researchers claim.

The simple act of smelling this treat may produce the same result, interestingly.

One research showed that smelling 85 percent dark chocolate lowered both hunger and starvation hormones just as much as consuming it.

However, to investigate the effects of dark chocolate on feelings of fullness, further studies are required.

Eating dark chocolate or even just smelling it will help suppress the appetite and cravings for sweets.

8. Feed a little ginger

Many health advantages have been related to ginger. That involves decreases in nausea, pain in the joints, inflammation, and levels of blood sugar.

Interestingly, recent research adds another advantage to the list: reducing hunger.

One research showed that the breakfast of 2 grams of ginger powder dissolved in hot water decreased the hunger participants felt after the meal.

This study, however, was limited, and further research is needed in humans before firm conclusions can be drawn.

Ginger will help reduce feelings of hunger, but to validate this effect, more research is required.

9. Spice your meals up

Ginger may not be the only spice that decreases hunger.

The effects of capsaicin, found in hot peppers, and capsiate, found in sweet peppers, have been investigated in a recent study.

These compounds were discovered to help alleviate hunger and improve feelings of fullness.

What's more, the heat generation potential of these

compounds can also increase the number of calories burned after a meal.

These impacts have not, however, been seen in all studies and remain minimal. In reality, people who consume these items will sometimes build a tolerance for the effects.

Compounds found in hot and sweet peppers can help reduce hunger and increase fullness, but further studies are needed.

10. Eat on Smaller Plates

Reducing your dinnerware's size will help you minimize your meal portions unconsciously. Without feeling hungry, this is likely to help you eat less food.

Interestingly, even the most conscious eater can be fooled by this effect.

Research, for example, found that when given larger bowls, even nutrition experts unintentionally served themselves 31 percent more ice cream.

Research has shown that you're likely to eat more without noticing it when you have more on your plate.

Without increasing your hunger stimuli, eating from smaller plates will make you unconsciously eat less.

11. Using a Bigger Fork

The size of your eating utensils can have a huge impact on the amount of food you need to feel whole.

One research showed that people who used bigger forks consumed 10 percent less with a smaller fork than those consuming their meals.

The researchers hypothesized that tiny forks might give individuals the impression that they are not making much progress in satisfying their hunger, leading them to eat more.

Of note, it does not seem to extend this effect to the scale of all utensils. Larger serving spoons will increase the food consumed during a meal by up to 14.5%.

Until reaching fullness, the use of larger forks can help reduce the amount of food required.

12. Exercise

Exercise is believed to decrease the activation of brain regions associated with cravings for food, which can lead to a lower desire to eat.

It may also decrease levels of starvation hormones while increasing feelings of fullness.

Research indicates that aerobic exercise and resistance are equally successful in affecting the levels of hormones and the size of a meal consumed after exercise.

Both aerobic and resistance exercises will help increase the hormones of fullness and decrease appetite and calories.

13. Lose fat from the body around your middle

A hormone that affects appetite and energy balance is neuropeptide Y (NPY).

It is known that higher NPY levels raise appetite and can even alter the number of calories that you store as fat.

Interestingly, researchers have found that body fat can increase the production of NPY, particularly the form found around your organs.

Because of this, losing weight around the core will help minimize the level of appetite and hunger.

14. Sleep Enough

It can also help alleviate hunger and protect against weight gain by having adequate quality sleep.

Study shows that too little sleep can increase hunger and appetite by up to 24% and decrease some fullness hormone levels by up to 26%.

The study also shows that people who sleep less than seven hours a night rated their fullness levels as 26 percent lower after breakfast.

It is worth noting that several studies also link short sleep, typically described as less than six hours per night, with an increased risk of obesity of up to 55 percent.

It is possible that having at least seven hours of sleep a night will decrease your levels of hunger during the day.

15. Reduce tension

It is understood that excess stress increases levels of the hormone cortisol.

Although the results can differ between people, it is commonly assumed that high cortisol increases food cravings and the desire to eat.

Stress can also reduce peptide YY (PYY) levels, a fullness hormone.

In a recent experiment, as compared to a non-stressful version of the same task, participants ate an average of 22 percent more calories after a stressful task.

It can not only help to curb hunger, but also reduce the risk of obesity and depression to find ways to reduce the stress levels.

Reducing your levels of stress will help minimize cravings, improve fullness, and even protect against depression and obesity.

16. Eat the Fats of Omega-3

Omega-3 fats, particularly those found in fish and algae oils, are capable of the levels of leptin, the fullness hormone.

When calories are restricted for weight loss, a diet rich in omega-3 fats can also improve fullness after meals.

These results have so far only been reported in participants who are overweight and obese. Further research is required to see if the same applies to lean individuals.

For overweight and obese people, omega-3 fats can help decrease appetite. In lean individuals, however, further study is required.

17. Opt for Snacks with Protein-Rich

Snacking is a matter of personal selection.

If it's part of your everyday routine, you might want to select high-protein snacks instead of high-fat ones.

High-protein snacks will increase feelings of fullness and decrease the following meal's overall calorie intake.

A high-protein yogurt, for example, more efficiently reduces appetite than high-fat crackers or a high-fat chocolate snack.

Compared with the other two choices, high-protein yogurt eaten in the afternoon can also help you consume about 100 fewer calories at dinner.

It is possible that consuming a protein-rich snack may decrease appetite and will prevent your next meal from overeating.

18. Visualize Eating the things you crave.

Picturing yourself indulging in the foods you enjoy most may potentially reduce your desire to eat them, according to some researchers.

In one experiment, before being granted access to a bowl of candy, 51 participants first imagined consuming either three or 33 M&Ms. Those who pictured eating more M&Ms, on average, consumed 60% less of the candy.

When they replicated the experiment using cheese instead of M&Ms, the researchers found the same effect.

The imagination exercise seems to trick your mind into thinking that you have already consumed the desired foods, greatly reducing the appetite for them.

It can reduce your desire to eat them by visualizing yourself consuming the foods you crave.

Hunger, which should not be overlooked, is an essential and natural warning.

Only a few easy ways to reduce your appetite and hunger between meals are the tips listed here.

If you've tried these things but still find that you're overly hungry, consider talking about your choices with a healthcare professional.

Chapter 10: LOVE YOURSELF WHEN LOSING WEIGHT

It seems a little counterintuitive to try to enjoy yourself when you lose weight. You work hard to improve your body, after all, so that must mean that you don't enjoy it the way it is, right? It doesn't have to be mutually exclusive to want to get better and embrace the body you have today.

In the sense of your overall health, start by thinking about your weight. That means extending your attention to include more than just the numbers on the scale, the way your jeans fit, and, yes, even what you see in the mirror.

You should be inspired, energized, and made to feel proud of yourself by embarking on a safe weight loss program. It also needs patience and time. For many, this can be a high order. Still, note, you are more likely to set reasonable goals when you start a weight loss journey from a position of self-love and acceptance and prepare for the little setbacks and disappointments that are a common stumbling block for many.

You will find some tips below to help you stay optimistic and true to yourself on the journey to maintaining a healthier weight.

TREAT EVERY DAY AS A NEW START.

Start each day by promising yourself that, no matter what happened yesterday, you will do the best you can. Thinking about every day as an opportunity for a new start will help you stop slipping into the negative self-talk trap that causes many individuals early in the process to give up on their weight loss goals.

GIVE A COMPLIMENT TO YOURSELF ONCE A DAY.

It may sound dumb, but it can help promote self-kindness (and restrict self-doubt, leading to self-loathing) to come naturally. Remembering what you love about yourself makes you want the best for your body, too, in the right mindset.

ACCEPT HOW YOU LOOK

Self-acceptance for the great variety of body shapes and sizes is a state of grace and respect. All of us are distinct, and who you are and what you look like is special; instead of concentrating on being someone else's idea of "great," note that your weight loss journey is about having better health.

FOCUS ON THE GIFTS THAT YOUR BODY GAVE YOU

It pushed you through your half marathon; it gave you two lovely girls. Without question, the body you might be down on has given you much potential and joy. A significant way of enjoying yourself as you lose weight is to revel in those memories and all that is still in store for you.

SET ATTAINABLE GOALS.

It's an easy road to disappointment and self-blaming to drop a dress size in time for your high school reunion in six days. Also, coming down on yourself in this way can lead to increased levels of the stress hormone cortisol, which has been shown to increase the amount of belly fat stored by the body, particularly in women.

A safer way to preserve your self-esteem and value your body's limits is to set a more attainable target, such as taking a new fitness class once a week or exchanging one sweet treat for a healthy alternative.

FEEL THE BENEFITS OF WORKOUTS

You know that one of the keys to good weight loss is exercise. What you may not know, though, is that physical activity in the brain triggers feel-good chemicals that elevate your mood. Research also indicates that those who exercise frequently appear to score their levels of self-esteem as higher than those who don't, as part of a weight-loss regimen.

If it's difficult to find the inspiration to work out, recruit a friend to exercise with you. Just as learning to love yourself as you lose weight is beneficial, there is no better cheerleader to take on your journey than someone who wants the best for you and reminds you daily of how good you are.

5 THINGS TO REMEMBER AFTER WEIGHT LOSS ABOUT BODY IMAGE

Most people believe that you feel better and happier after you lose weight, and you may be.

But adapting to new body size, no matter what the number on the scale suggests, will do a number on your self-esteem. You can no longer recognize yourself and face problems with your body, such as stretch marks or loose skin.

You can also fail to get recognition or compliments resulting from your loss of weight. One research, in particular, found that losing weight doesn't make you happier automatically.

Want a variety of exercise? The newest workouts from Aaptiv are now in the app.

It may also result in a higher risk of anxiety and depression.

Our specialists discuss how weight loss impacts the perception of the body and share their best tips for healthy acceptance of the body.

Your reasons for weight loss would affect how you feel afterward.

Weight loss normally happens to improve life patterns, according to Mayra Mendez, Ph.D., a psychotherapist at Providence Saint John's Child and Family Development Center.

Besides boost stamina, energy levels, and agility, this is to be healthier.

However, based on external pressure and idealized social expectations, people are often inspired to lose weight.

Or they want from others to obtain recognition and value. Body acceptance is more likely for the first form, but self-image appears to be more negative for the second.

"Erin Wathen, a food addiction specialist and holistic wellness and life coach, says:" Body image after weight loss can be very complicated.

Even an extra 15 pounds can be an excuse not to go for a big job or the reason why in our relationships we don't speak up for ourselves. We need to reconcile what that extra weight has done to us. It might have kept you safe, e.g., not having to go back after a breakup to the dating pool. Or because of your size, it served as a human shield from criticism of choices you made as a parent. We wouldn't have remained there as long as we did if anything about being a different weight was terrible. The key is to identify it, recognize it, and find a new process of thinking in order not to remain small in our own lives.

Weight loss will lead to a relationship with your body that is very positive.

"Let's start with the healthy," says Kelly Chase, the Aaptiv trainer.

"Weight loss will enhance the appearance of your body. In your new size, you can gain more faith, appreciate the effort you put into achieving your aim of weight loss and be motivated to make others feel comfortable and secure as well. I do believe that everyone should have a healthy relationship with their body, no matter their size, and embrace their curves beautifully. I have accepted my body a lot more now that I have lost unwanted weight on my weight loss journey. But I would continue to say positive affirmations every day when I was heavier, change my mindset and embrace my body for what it was, which helped retain as much of a positive mindset as possible.

Weight loss will promote a desire to take care of your body, look in the mirror and feel good about yourself, and identify more often with parts of your body that you like.

Also, Mendez says, it can strengthen healthy behaviors and validate feelings of achievement regarding your goals for weight loss.

But even though, mentally, you feel fine, the emotional side will tell a different story.

The challenge of looking good on the outside while suffering emotionally on the inside is understood firsthand by many people who have lost weight.

That's normal, says therapist Heidi McBain. It doesn't always help to hear affirmation for weight loss because it either confirms you were overweight before or highlights the physical versus the inside of you.

And if you continually compare your body to other people, or if it doesn't seem like you've lost enough weight, the dominant paradigm may be shameful, Mendez says.

That is because the picture of the body is perceptual, not physical. This suggests that you more see yourself as bigger, heavier, shorter, or stockier than you are even though you lose weight, she adds.

Chase says, "Weight loss doesn't always build a good body picture."

It may lead to loose skin, muscle loss or curves or booty gains, and stretch marks. An even bigger issue, such as fear of food or fear of eating too much and gaining weight again, may also be developed. To help you on your journey, it's best to surround yourself with supportive individuals, or even a wellness coach.

And you're surrounded by positivity and raising you by individuals, which can build a positive attitude.

Acceptance of the body has little to do with how much you weigh.

Devin Alexander, who has managed a 70-pound weight loss for over 20 years and now works as the chef for NBC's The Biggest Loser, says, "Weight loss is not at all a surefire road to body acceptance." She states that, due to drastic body dysmorphia, many individuals don't have a reasonable view of themselves.

I lost 70 pounds in my situation, was a size two, and was always thinking I wasn't attractive. After several broken plans, [this] landed me in Overeaters Anonymous because I couldn't find anything to wear,' Alexander says.

I always thought I'd be able to walk into a department store if I was a size two, put something on, and look amazing. Instead, though I still had big hips, I started feeling girlie, and my chest and curves were disappearing. I knew my body is best at a size four when I got my head straight and gained a couple of pounds back. Not extremely lean, but fit.

The bottom line, Mendez acknowledges, is that acceptance of the body allows each person to go on an individual journey. To challenge negative expectations needs more than weight loss.

You will begin to see your worth by recognizing that you deserve and have a right to happiness and contentment, regardless of your weight or how your body looks.

"No matter their size, body dysmorphia can affect everyone," Chase says. I have known many women who either lose weight or are still slim, who have unrealistic or negative body photos of themselves, and believe that they are 'fat.' The mind needs to be changed at this point. From negative to positive self-talk, you transition your mind.

You can use these ideas to get back on the right track if you're struggling.

The hard work, holding the weight off, often starts after we have hit our target size or weight, "Chase says."

"Therefore, it would do wonders for your self-esteem to surround yourself with inspiring and compassionate friends and family or even a new group of friends. [It will] facilitate healthy acceptance of the body.'

1. According to our experts, here are some tips for body acceptance following weight loss.
2. Maintain a rational view of the objectives you set for yourself by focusing on them.
3. Write out and say regular optimistic affirmations.
4. Believe you're entitled to be proud of your efforts.
5. Initiate a regimen of meditation to make you feel more concentrated and grounded.
6. To see the improvement, take pictures of yourself.
7. See yourself as an entire human, not just a person who has lost weight.
8. Keep a journal of appreciation to reflect on all the good of your life.
9. Give yourself time to adapt to the physical, mental, and psychological changes associated with weight loss.
10. Dress up or recruit a stylist for your new body to help you find clothes that make you feel amazing.
11. Share with others about your journey.
12. Speak to a psychologist for assistance with body image distortion or unhealthy ways of thought.

I began to wear a baby image of myself in a locket ring as part of my healing, with the promise that I would never say something to myself that I wouldn't say to a small child, "Alexander shares."

It's awesome how much we mean to ourselves. I compelled myself to act as I do to someone else with love for myself, which changed my attitude tremendously.

Talk to a professional.

Pay attention to red flags that may suggest that you need

further assistance on your journey to accepting the body.

Mendez says these often include suicidal thoughts and emotions that are debilitating or paralyzing, isolation from friends and family, lack of grooming or self-care, neglecting duties or responsibilities, or increased misuse of drugs.

Chase says that looking back, she had a lot of guilt overeating and gaining weight. It wasn't until she put her faith in a health coach that she resolved a fear of embracing her body and developing a more healthy relationship with food.

To support you in the fitness path, Aaptiv has top trainers. Check out the workouts we have in the app for fitness.

"Alexander says," We're referring to accountants and financial advisors and arborists and lawyers and so many other experts who have learned subjects we haven't.

Why is it so hard for so many people to turn to trainers or counselors or other personal experts? It takes courage to realize that you do not know everything and might profit from the experience of another person. If, as Nike would say, you're struggling, just do it.'

Chapter 11: UNDERSTANDING HYPNOTHERAPY GASTRIC BAND

A method used to help you lose weight is gastric band hypnotherapy. A hypnotherapist uses this strategy to communicate to your subconscious that you have had a gastric band fitted around your stomach. Considered to be a non-invasive alternative to surgery for weight loss, without the possible side effects, a hypnotic gastric band can have many of the positive effects.

One type of weight loss surgery that is sometimes seen as a last resort is a conventional gastric band. The band physically limits how much food you can consume by fitting a band around the upper portion of your stomach, facilitating weight loss in many situations. Research has, however, shown that in the months and years following surgery, patients undergoing a physical gastric band face a variety of complications, including the possibility of slipping or eroding the band.

For those that have struggled with sustainable weight loss, lifestyle changes, and weight-related problems, the often dramatic and enduring loss of weight that follows many gastric band procedures can be very enticing. It needs no surgery to get a 'virtual gastric band' installed, also known as gastric band hypnotherapy.

A hypnotherapist will enable you, on an unconscious level, to feel that you have had a physical operation by interacting with your subconscious and that your stomach has decreased in size. No surgery or drug is used, making it an option that is safer and painless. We're going to discuss how this approach works, what it means, and how it can work for you.

What is a gastric band?

An adjustable silicone brace used in surgery for weight loss is a gastric band. To build a small pouch above the unit, the band is located around the upper section of your stomach. This reduces the amount of food in your stomach that can be processed, making it impossible to consume large quantities.

A gastric band is one of the three weight-loss operations most widely provided, available via private surgery, or for those with a BMI of 40 or more who meet particular requirements for an NHS operation. A gastric band's biggest advantage is long-term, permanent weight loss. It's also necessary to change your diet, exercise regularly, and attend post-surgery follow-up appointments to obtain advice and help as required for you to see the benefits.

The purpose of a gastric band is to reduce the amount of food a person can consume physically, allowing them to feel full to promote weight loss after consuming very little. It is the final resort for most people who have this surgery after attempting other weight loss strategies. Fitting a gastric band comes with complications, like any surgery.

Some of the risks include if you have a physical gastric band:

- The band slips out of place. This can lead to nausea, vomiting, and heartburn. To readjust or remove the band, further surgery may be required.
- A leak in the gut. There is a small risk that food may leak into your tummy following a gastric bypass or gastric sleeve (another type of gastric band), causing a severe infection that may require antibiotics and surgery to fix any damage.
- A blocked stomach. Blockages may cause vomiting, tummy pain, difficulty swallowing, and bowel movement disorders. Blockages would have to be cleared by a specialist.
- Malnutrition. After weight loss surgery, consuming the right amount of vitamins and minerals can become an issue, which ensures that many would have to take supplements for life to prevent the risks of malnutrition.

For 12-18 months post-surgery, women who have had a physical gastric band, sleeve, or bypass are also advised to prevent pregnancy.

But how do gastric physical bands vary from gastric band hypnosis? And can a gastrointestinal virtual band have the same benefits?

Hypnosis of the Gastric Band

Gastric band hypnosis can be used, without the complications that come with surgery, to help people lose weight. Many hypnotherapists use a two-pronged approach. They first look at the root cause of your emotional eating to recognize it.

WHAT IS EMOTIONAL NUTRITION?

A common but unhealthy way to cope with difficult feelings or emotions may be emotional eating. When you are frustrated or depressed, or rely on food as a treat or reward for a difficult week, to motivate yourself, or even as a fallback when you are bored, if you find yourself looking for food, these may all be indicators that you are using food to help improve your mood. This can lead to feelings of guilt, embarrassment, and even a pattern of poor eating habits over time that can lead to problems with eating, disordered eating, and physical health issues.

Using hypnosis, a hypnotherapist may enable you to recall long-forgotten food-related memories that might now subconsciously influence you. They will also help you identify patterns, responses, or habits that you may not know you've been doing. Before beginning gastric band hypnotherapy, discussing and identifying any unhealthy thinking patterns concerning food may be beneficial.

Next, the virtual gastric band procedure will be carried out by your hypnotherapist. Gastric band hypnotherapy is intended to indicate that you have undergone an operation to implant a gastric band at a subconscious level. The intention is for your body to respond to this suggestion by making you feel fuller faster than having the actual surgery.

Compared to diets, having a virtual gastric band is intended to help you make major changes in your lifestyle. Hypnotherapy will help you take the first steps in making meaningful progress by identifying and resolving root problems, helping you to understand causes, and engaging with your subconscious to help you feel fuller for longer.

Diets do not seem to cope with the necessary lasting changes in lifestyle, such as a positive long-term shift in eating habits and food attitude. Many diet plans are temporary, either because they are too restrictive or they fully deprive us of our favorite foods, which can be difficult to manage on an ongoing basis.

These regimes can be adhered to in the short term, but in the long run, they do not perform so well. Many diets can make us more concerned with food and eating by causing us to count calories or actively measure portion size or even completely omit food types. This can take the fun of eating out and lead us to want more of those foods, and it can begin a diet-overeat / binge loop.

-Hypnotherapist Becca Teers discusses why weight-loss diets do not work.

HOW GASTRIC BAND HYPNOSIS PERFORMS

A hypnotherapist can place you in a state of hypnosis using calming techniques. Your subconscious is more open to suggestions in this comfortable state. Hypnotherapists make recommendations to your subconscious at this stage. This recommendation is that you get a physical band fitted with gastric band hypnotherapy.

The mind is strong, so your behavior will adjust accordingly if your subconscious follows these suggestions. Usually, along with the 'fitting' of the virtual gastric band, motivation and attitude interventions will be made to help you stick to this lifestyle change.

Many therapists can also teach strategies of self-hypnosis so that you can strengthen the work you've done after the session. It is also always recommended to educate yourself on diet and exercise to encourage physical health and well-being.

Unhealthy diet relationships

It might also be worth contemplating your relationship with food if you contemplate weight-related surgery or hypnotherapy alternatives. Simply concentrating on the overall objective of weight loss may also ignore the underlying problems of an unhealthy relationship with food that can impact you in various aspects of your life, including impacting your self-confidence, self-esteem, triggering feelings of anxiety or remorse, or even keeping you back in social or work-related circumstances.

The eating problem does not have a single 'look.' It can affect someone in any number of different ways, at any age. It's important to talk with your GP if you're worried that your eating habits may affect your overall health and well-being.

What to expect: having a gastric virtual band

An initial appointment will be your first meeting with the hypnotherapist to explore what you expect to learn from hypnotherapy. This is a chance to chat about your past attempts at weight loss, your eating habits, your health conditions, and your general food attitude. This data will give the psychiatrist a better picture of what will benefit and whether any other forms of therapy should be taken into consideration or not.

Note: it's important to seek advice from your doctor if you have any health issues related to your weight.

The operation itself is intended to imitate surgery of the gastric band, to assist your subconscious in assuming that it happened. The sounds and smells of an operating theatre would be introduced by many hypnotherapists to make the experience more real. By getting you into a profoundly relaxed state, also known as hypnosis, your therapist will begin. At all times, you will be conscious of what is happening and will be in charge.

The therapist will talk you through the operation until you are in a hypnotic state. From being placed under the anesthetic to making the first incision, fitting the band itself, and fixing up the wound, they can describe step by step what happens in surgery. To reassure the subconscious that what is being said is happening to you, the sounds and smells of an operating theatre will increase the experience.

During the process, other ideas may be implemented to improve self-confidence. Your hypnotherapist can teach you some self-hypnosis techniques once the treatment is complete, to help you stay on track at home.

Some hypnotherapists may recommend returning for follow-up appointments to help track the performance of the virtual gastric band and make any changes. This occurs as individuals also mount the physical band. For others, as part of a long-term weight-loss strategy, maintaining hypnotherapy sessions may be helpful. This encourages the hypnotherapist to work with you to fix the underlying diet and self-esteem problems.

Hypnosis of the gastric band can be part of a program of weight control that discusses diet and exercise patterns. For those pursuing weight loss, it is the combination of modifying behaviors in both the body and mind that is often most effective.

How am I going to feel afterward?

Recognizing when you're mentally full can be challenging for those who over-eat. Sometimes we eat, ignoring whether or not we are physically hungry, simply for taste or warmth. To cultivate good eating habits, learning to understand the physical sensations of being hungry and full is beneficial.

With most individuals reporting a sense of relaxation as they come out of hypnosis, the treatment should be a fun and calming experience.

Can hypnotherapy for the gastric band work for me?

For those seeking hypnotherapy for the first time, a common question is: will it work for me? It's not, unfortunately, a straightforward case of yes or no; it's ultimately up to you. Hypnotherapy helps people with a variety of problems, but when it comes to changing behaviors, it is especially helpful. It is also effective, for this reason, in helping people develop healthier eating habits and lose weight. Nevertheless, just like any other lifestyle improvements, your complete dedication will be needed.

No type of weight loss is assured of producing precise outcomes from surgery to diets. Similarly, the effects of gastric band hypnotherapy, as with any type of hypnosis, rely on you entering the process with an open mind, as well as being ready and willing to make changes.

If you trust in the process and your therapist, you are more likely to make sustainable modifications and get what you want from gastric band hypnotherapy. It is important to be relaxed and trust your hypnotherapist. This is why it is recommended that you take time in your field to study hypnotherapists and find out more about them, how they function, and what their qualifications include. Before you begin, you should arrange to meet with them to guarantee that you feel comfortable with them.

Gastric band hypnosis should work for you if you are dedicated to making a lifestyle change, believe in the process, and trust your hypnotherapist.

Is a gastric virtual band the best option for me?

It will rely on several different factors, whether a virtual gastric band is right for you or not. It can be a perfect alternative to conventional surgery for certain individuals. Others can find it to be a useful instrument for making positive changes in lifestyles and sustainable weight loss. It's important to note that there are several different strategies and choices open to you, whatever your situation is.

5 STUFF YOU DIDN'T HEAR ABOUT HYPNOTHERAPY GASTRIC BAND

The first thing that crosses my mind is that I should warn you that hypnotherapy for the gastric band is not for everyone; what I say is that for everyone, it's not effective. Those who genuinely want to improve their weight, eating habits, and food relationships are the most active patients. Many looking for a crutch or just a helping hand so that they don't have to apply themselves are not likely to be as successful in the longer term. For those with the right attitude, hypnotic suggestion works better, but this does not mean that gastric band hypnotherapy does not work for you; each case is evaluated for suitability on its own merits.

Please feel free to check out some video testimonials and reviews from a colleague based in Australia to try to demonstrate impartiality about the procedure.

Below, I will talk about five stuff you didn't know about gastric band hypnotherapy to try to figure out what you do understand.

You don't have a fitted gastric band,

It seems a straightforward point to cover, but I've had some calls from individuals misunderstanding the practice of gastric band hypnotherapy with the actual private or NHS medical treatment. Hypnoband is the most general practice of hypnotherapy for the gastric band and does not require surgery.

Hypnotherapy is a non-invasive type of hypnotherapy for weight loss that utilizes suggestions and cognitive behavioral therapy to achieve the desired results. There is no need for a hospital, doctor, or nurse to come, perfect if you have any of the above fears.

Is it going to work for me?

Hypnotherapy for the gastric band is contingent on you. In your mind and heart, you need to be completely committed to losing weight. This approach is not for those who are seeking to "take care of something else." The secret to your success is YOU!

Candidates must be prepared to improve their eating habits and lifestyle overall. If more than one person in your household is acceptable for the counseling, consider this if that person is not prepared to change their habits. If you are constantly around causes and reminders to consume big or inappropriate meals, this might directly affect your findings.

It will work for you if you are serious about losing weight.

Is it assured that Gastric Band Hypnotherapy will help me lose weight?

Due to any number of variables that may influence the outcome of the treatment or practice, no medical carry any clear assurance of outcome. One thing that we can confirm is that gastric band hypnotherapy is not going to have any medical side effects.

You have to note that the results are based on the person with some sort of hypnosis, stopping smoking, fear of heights or spiders, that's YOU! If you are not 100 percent committed, no form of hypnotherapy will work.

You have to know that the mind is a very complex and strong

organ, and you can arm yourself with the requisite instruments to change your old eating habits for good by having gastric band hypnotherapy. The treatment aims to help you improve your attitude and lifestyle, helping you to improve your relationship with food and lose weight.

What do I expect from my treatment course?

Hypnotherapy care of the gastric band consists of an evaluation session as well as multiple hour-long therapy sessions. To help you "top up" the treatment further down the road, we also facilitate this with a CD or MP3 recording.

Before dealing with any therapy, a successful therapist would have a complete breakdown of your food and medical history. You will be exposed to hypnosis during the first session, a state of heightened learning, where you will also feel very relaxed and calm.

You will be introduced to the gastric band hypnotherapy during the following sessions, and your hypnotherapist will work with you to "suit" the virtual gastric band for optimum impact.

The later sessions will address your interaction with food and your eating habits.

What would it cost?

Sadly, around the board, there are no fixed rates. The more successful your therapist has been in his work, the more they can fee, as their arguments can be backed up, and outcomes are shown.

Depending on your situation, how you might probably handle it is to compare the prices you are quoted vs. the quoted prices of medical gastric bands that I have seen advertised in London above £5,950.

I would assume that to cover your appraisal, care, and

subsequent MP3 or CD support services, you would fairly expect to pay a quarter to a third of that amount. For several occasions, you may wish to complete your gastric band hypnotherapy treatment far further down the road.

Would you like to lose weight?

Thousands of people feel the same way as you do right now. The celebrations added a few extra pounds and the drinking sessions appear to have continued from there. Christmas was and is gone.

But you know, deep down, you just aren't pleased about what's going on, and you want to adjust.

So far, diets may not have worked for you, but you're willing to try something that can give you the optimistic edge you need to control your food cravings.

Here is How Hypnosis of the Gastric Band Functions.

Instead of making the stomach narrower and re-routing the intestines as is done with gastric bypass, surgical gastric banding entails inserting a tube-like ring around the stomach, limiting the amount of food consumed safely and restricting the digestive tract's development. So that the rate of weight loss is regulated, the band can be made tighter or looser.

In the protection and comfort of your head, gastric band hypnosis guides you through planning, surgery, and healthy post-op living.

The old thoughts and feelings used to sidetrack you from your goals for weight loss will begin to be remembered. Only now can you have fresh, safer ways of reacting to those old behaviors and patterns.

At this point, you might think something like, "Yeah, in a stage show, people dance like Elvis, but when the show is done, they come out of it." After the hypnosis session terminates, how does this work? Let's together discuss stage hypnosis vs. gastric band hypnosis.

Stage shows use hypnosis as a way to impress an audience. Usually, the people on stage are volunteers who know what they're in for or are interested and eager to have some fun.

For the background of the display, the recommendations they obey are given only and are omitted when they are taken out of hypnosis.

The use of post-hypnotic feedback is one distinction between stage hypnosis and therapeutic hypnosis. Sometimes, before waking their volunteers, a successful stage hypnotist can provide post-hypnotic tips for energy, well-being, and a great night's sleep.

In the deeper stages of trance, where the conscious mind is less active, post-hypnotic suggestions are made. Post-hypnotic advice given at the required depth in therapeutic hypnosis help you to make the changes you want to look normal because they are.

Should I have a memory that never happened to me?

Have you ever woken up from a deep sleep, not knowing if it was a dream or if it happened? It felt genuine, emotionally intense, but it wasn't.

Have you ever had a vision that shaped how you feel about someone else, or changed your normal method of decision-making?

This very normal capacity of your brain to bridge your dream world with your waking world is used through gastric band hypnosis.

- Can gastric band hypnosis still function if I remember I haven't had surgery?
- Think of the last good film you've seen.
- Did you know it was just a movie?

- That those individuals were not actual individuals, just actors pretending?
- That the stuff that happened never happened, or at least did not happen at the moment and did not happen to you in particular?
- And did you get involved emotionally, anyway?

That is referred to as a suspension of unbelief. You allowed yourself to acknowledge the experiences presented as real and reacted in kind within the boundaries of the theatre.

On a conscious level, you will know that you have not undergone a surgical operation. Your adherence to the method of gastric band hypnosis ensures you want to believe and live as if you had it. That conviction primes your subconscious mind to consider pre-op, surgery, and post-op treatment suggestions.

Am I going to feel like I've had an operation? While gastric band hypnosis uses light or local Hypno-anesthesia, it is not unusual for individuals to smell antiseptic, experience a tugging sensation afterward with the sutures or a small amount of abdominal tenderness. As the body adapts to the changes it perceives, we suggest you take it easy the next day.

Does having hypnosis of the gastric band mean I'll never have to think again about diet and exercise?

For certain individuals, this is not a decision that you make once, and it works forever.

Hypnosis of the Gastric Band is a severe commitment. The more you treat it as surgery for the gastric band, the more successful it will be. You can always have free can, and no hypnosis will take it away from you and the desire to make unhealthy choices.

For the rest of your life, genuinely safe living comes from the commitment you make to yourself every day.

BASIC AND ADVANCED VIRTUAL GASTRIC BAND WEIGHT LOSS PROGRAMS

Since not everyone deals with the same problems, MindOverMatter provides two different Virtual Gastric Band Weight Loss Programs. While some know very well that they eat for emotional reasons, others put on weight after having a baby because, or for other reasons, their work or home situation has changed.

Both these programs for weight loss are about improving your relationship with food to live a lifestyle comfortably, and naturally, were listening to your body is the most important thing you can do. Only in smaller amounts can you eat whatever you want. In reality, dieting is something you used to do. There is no dieting. You don't feel deprived without dieting, there is no obsession with food, and cravings become less and less.

Basic Virtual Weight Loss

Mainly targeted to those who have put on weight due to pregnancy, shift work, travel, or some other cause for which it does not have an essential emotional aspect. This is not the emphasis, although there are methods within this curriculum to control emotional eating. Sometimes, but not always, those with a smaller amount of weight to lose can choose this program.

This program consists of 4 sessions over 10/12 weeks in clinics. Each session is between 45 minutes and 1.5 hours long.

A basic audio support download will be given for you to use in between sessions. These will enhance and improve the work of the clinic and allow for the strengthening and creation of new neural pathways within your brain. The mind works and learns by repetition, and while it takes three lots of 21 days to change a habit, as you move through the program, you will experience changes in actions, emotions, and thoughts.

You will be taught lots of new strategies during each session and provided tools to boost the clinic experience and support you on your journey. Elaine also offers support between sessions via email and phone if you ever need assistance.

Virtual Weight Loss

Mainly for emotional purposes, targeted to those who know why they eat. You have probably struggled all your life with your weight. For emotional reasons, like boredom, tension, irritation, rage, anxiety, joy, and excitement, you should feed. When you were younger, you may recall the food being used to reward or make you feel better. You do not have a memory of it at all; you just know that you can't manage it. You might eat the wrong stuff, or you might eat too much, or you might eat a combination of both.

This curriculum takes a hard look at why you eat and requires eight sessions spanning 16/18 weeks. Four of these sessions are a blend of talk therapy and work on hypnosis/energy. Four are focused on hypnoanalysis that enables Elaine to dig into the subconscious part of your mind where all the thoughts and emotions reside.

You will be granted two unique downloads of audio support to be used in between sessions. This will reinforce and expand the work of the clinic and allow for the strengthening and development of new neural pathways within the brain. The mind operates by repetition, and the audio shifts the present, unhelpful habits over time and generates new desirable habits.

To help you on this journey, you will also be presented with a wide range of tools and strategies to strengthen clinical work while building trust, confidence, and belief in yourself.

How does it function?

The subconscious is unaware of the distinction between actual and imagined.

I persuade your mind at the first session that you have a gastric band attached to the top of your stomach and that you should eat just half as much as when you first came into my clinic. It is a non-surgical technique that retrains the mind to be content with smaller amounts of food using the power of hypnosis. It changes how you think about food and gives outcomes that are very healthy and very predictable. After a certain amount of food consumption, the hypnosis convinces the brain that the stomach is full, and there is no need for more food. It's NOT a diet-we realize that diets only work in the short term; it's a life program. You can consume anything you want with the Interactive Weight Loss Program, but you will find yourself consuming smaller portions and usually healthy foods. And you're not going to feel deprived, unhappy or hungry, because it's not a diet. You'll probably be shocked by how easy it is to change your habits, and all you have is a long-term solution to your weight problem.

Both programs follow a method in which, through suggestions, pattern interrupts, imagery, and awareness, I create continuity from one week to the next to direct your mind towards the life you want, the individual you want to be. You begin to believe that you can do this, that you can accomplish your objectives by building your confidence by helping you to take back power by enabling you to link to that calm and comfortable part of your mind. At this point, it is important to remember that I will not make you do something you do not want to do and that you are the one in charge, while I am your guide.

We go through hypnoanalysis in the advanced curriculum, which is about uncovering the core illusion that you began eating all those years ago for emotional reasons. When did this begin? Why has it begun? We are only able to do this by using well-established hypnoanalytic techniques. When you become aware of where these feelings originated from, the next step is to realize what's around them and why, and then eventually overcome them by release and reframing. During the initial session, Elaine goes into greater detail about this process.

How can you produce the best results? To put 100 percent effort into this program, you make a promise to yourself. All of the time, those who make this effort succeed! "Without change, there's no change" If you do as you've always done, you get what you always get

We now realize, on a final note, that our thoughts and emotions can alter the structure and function of our brain and that we can change old obsolete habits and beliefs for the habits and beliefs we want today by rewiring (changing the neural pathways). The science of neuroplasticity has provided us with proof that by using the power of our minds, we only need to know how to choose to transform, alter, and evolve.

"It's all up to you now, and know that if you want to, you will completely" Live a Life That Counts.

THE VIRTUAL GASTRIC BAND HISTORY

Sheila Grainger, a clinical hypnotherapist about five years ago, came across a newspaper report about some people in Spain experimenting on the idea of using a weight-loss device for virtual gastric bands to lose weight. Sheila, who ran a good clinic in Yorkshire, was fascinated by this article and wanted to see if this idea had any merit. To see how successful it would be, she decided to run a trial and provided an invitation for volunteers to participate in the free trial and had little trouble achieving the numbers needed. She took on 25 volunteers and saw them in a group setting, of various shapes, sizes, age ranges, and gender. Since the care was not tailored, she envisaged possibly only a 40 percent success rate, assuming that its efficacy might be diminished through community therapy.

The advantages of Hypnotherapy in the Virtual Gastric Band

> ➤ This is NOT a diet to make you feel poor or hungry.
> ➤ No side effects or risks occur.

- ➢ Virtual gastric banding contributes to lasting improvements in the pattern of eating
- ➢ Compared to surgery or other diet items, the program is economical.
- ➢ If you are 5 kg or 50 kg overweight, it is successful.
- ➢ After your first session, you will note a transition.
- ➢ Eighty-three percent of this initiative gets results, and that is after two years.
- ➢ This will be the last time you spend cash on weight loss.
- ➢ You get back your health; then you get back your life.
- ➢ Establish a balanced relationship with food
- ➢ You can eat whatever you want, only in smaller quantities.
- ➢ You learn various techniques to cope with your feelings.
- ➢ How the services are coordinated

Basic Virtual Weight Loss

Due to pregnancy, shift work, travel, or some other cause that does not have a major emotional aspect, tailored to those who have put on weight. For more detail, see below), followed by the initial review session.

In a stressed-out mentality that has recently been transformed to your dinner plate? Meditation is a fantastic way to get your body and mind back on track, and it can involve a path to weight loss.

It's easy to establish less than desirable eating habits and an unhealthy relationship with food when you're under a lot of stress. You will find harmony with food through meditation and help bring 2020 behind you. Ok, here's how.

Chapter 12: HOW DOES MEDITATION RELATE TO FOOD AND WEIGHT LOSS

Meditation is a calming practice to calm your mind and redirect them. It's also a way of raising the consciousness of yourself and your climate. Mindfulness is a form of meditation that allows you to understand your physical sensations and emotions.

Since meditation is a way of generating consciousness, stress, or emotional eating may help it. This may be in the form of conscientious feeding.

What is eating with mindfulness?

Have you ever had such a wonderful-looking meal, but you thought you were so starving that without even enjoying it, you scarfed it down? You weren't aware of your meal in this situation.

To be conscious of the full experience while feeding, mindful eating uses mindfulness. The foundations of mindful eating include remembering that:

> ➢ How easily you eat
> ➢ What you drink
> ➢ How certain foods cause you to feel
> ➢ Using your senses to feel food color, smell, taste, and textures.
> ➢ Why are you eating (are you eating out of hunger, fear, or feelings?)
> ➢ Your cravings and what's behind them
> ➢ The signs that tell you that you are complete
> ➢ How to handle food-related shame and anxiety
> ➢ What to eat for good

Tips for eating with mindfulness

Start concentrating on one meal a day to incorporate mindful eating, and keep these tips in mind:

> • Eat slowly and enjoy the meal. Don't hurry!

- Chew carefully. Don't take two bites and swallow and taste the spice.
- Get rid of distractions, such as your mobile phone or TV.
- Aim to eat in silence.
- Concentrate on what you eat and how it makes you feel.
- When you are finished, stop feeding.
- Tell yourself why you eat. Are you hungry physically or hungry emotionally?

What about eating intuitively?

An anti-diet that teaches you to trust the hunger signals of your body is a form of mindful eating, intuitive eating. When it comes to your body and what you will eat, you are the determining factor and the expert. And, you just know the signs of your thirst.

You are weighing the reasons behind eating as an intuitive eater. Are you tired, irritable, and your nutrients need to be replenished? Or are you depressed, lonely, and yearning for food to comfort your feelings?

WEIGHT LOSS MEDITATION BENEFITS

Meditation and healthy eating will help you enjoy and appreciate the journey of your food, which can have tremendous benefits for weight loss in turn. Here are several ways you can lose weight with meditation.

Loss of Sustainable Weight

Meditation was found to improve eating habits and be a validated tool for weight loss in a 2017 study of previous mindfulness meditation research. Many who used meditation for mindfulness were more likely to hold the weight off, too.

Meditation on mindfulness can be broken down into three sections to help maintain weight loss:

1. The location where you are
2. What you put in your body
3. The way you feel at the moment
4. Reduce tension and control it

Research in 2011 showed that mindful eating would help improve eating habits and decrease stress, contributing to weight loss. We make less time for healthy behaviors and decisions while we are anxious.

Stress makes it more difficult to lose weight and releases the cortisol hormone, which has been associated with causing those comfort food cravings. Stress also raises the amount of insulin, making it more difficult for the body to burn off the food.

Help prevent binge and unhealthy emotional eating

By improving your eating habits, mindful eating will help you lose weight and relieve stress. When something bad happens, or you eat a pizza, this will help you stop searching for sweets.

A big consideration for weight loss is changing how you feel about food. To help build self-control around food, you have to put those negative feelings about food behind you and become completely aware of the positive emotions.

In the past, the effectiveness of your long-term weight loss improves when you quit such harmful eating habits.

Having more sleep

Meditation practice will help you learn to redirect the racing thoughts that keep you awake in the evening. Studies have shown that those who were studied using mindfulness meditation in randomized research fell asleep earlier and slept longer than those who didn't.

Feel less shame because of food

When it comes to food, guilt and shame have no place.

The worst thing you can do at the moment is to be judgmental about yourself. Recognize your emotions and habits of behavior. You have to forgive yourself for the minor mishaps along the way as well. You won't slip back into the loop over and over until you forgive yourself. But if it does ... pause, and again forgive.

For meditation on mindfulness, take it one step at a time to understand these patterns.

How to Start to Meditate

Now that you know how meditation can aid your path to weight loss, how the heck are you going to start?

When you start, allow yourself just 10 minutes a day to concentrate on meditating. To concentrate on yourself, you'll have to decide to realign your components.

For a balanced relationship with food, the same goes. Work to release any shame you may have about food with kindness and practice knowledge of what you put in your body and why.

Without any distractions, find a peaceful spot. You can sit or lie down (whichever is more comfortable). Make sure your back is straight if you're seated, your hands on your lap, your neck relaxed, and your head slightly tucked in.

To start meditating, here are some steps:

1. Take a deep breath, hold it for a few seconds, and exhale slowly.
2. Repeat for about 20 seconds to ensure that your gaze is gentle or that your eyes are closed and that you breathe in through your nose and out through your mouth.
3. Continue to breathe naturally.
4. Observe your stance, scan the body, and identify the senses.
5. For 5 to 10 minutes, concentrate on your breath.
6. Think about why this is where you are and watch your breath.

7. Enable it to free your body.
8. Be mindful of where you are and what you are going to do next.

For weight loss, guided meditation applications

Need guided meditation help? Here are some applications that will direct you with support. Many of these apps are free and offer premium content that is paid for.

THE MINDFULNESS APP

This app has driven meditations and data on how to get started. From 3 to 30 minutes, both quiet and synchronized meditations can be used. It also has customized choices, including a meditation journal and reminders, to suit every lifestyle.

HeadSpace

For all things quiet, Headspace is an app. With directed meditation and mindfulness exercises, with its sleep music tracks and nature soundscapes, it's perfect for daytime and even nighttime. This program will encourage you to learn to create your meditation.

Calm

The Calm app is known for many methods, such as breathing exercises, a meditation on mindful walking, and exercises for relaxing. It also has portions of Sleep Stories with famous actors reading bedtime stories to you.

Relaxation and Meditation Pro

To keep meditation simple but efficient, this easy-to-follow app is built. To alleviate tension, sleep easier, and improve your self-esteem, you will find meditation.

In some ways, meditation can be used. It is a way of becoming aware of your needs and ambitions and eventually becoming aware of what you put in your body. It will teach you how to build mindful eating habits and help you on your journey towards weight loss.

Chapter 13: THE PLANET'S 20 MOST WEIGHT LOSS FRIENDLY FOODS

We can receive a small commission if you purchase anything through a connection on this page. Only how it works.

Not all calories are equal in life.

In your body, various foods go through various metabolic pathways.

They can have vastly different effects on your appetite, hormones, and how many calories you burn.

Here are the science-supported 20 most weight-loss-friendly foods on earth.

1. Whole Eggs

Once they were hated for being high in cholesterol, whole eggs made a comeback.

Since a high intake of eggs boosts some people's levels of "bad" LDL-cholesterol, if you need to lose weight, they are one of the best foods to eat. They're high in fat and protein, and they're very satisfying.

One study of 30 women who were overweight found that instead of bagels, consuming eggs for breakfast improved feelings of fullness (satiety) and made participants eat less for the next 36 hours.

Another eight-week study found that compared to bagels, eggs for breakfast improved weight loss on a calorie-restricted diet.

Eggs are also extremely rich in nutrients and can help you get all the nutrients on a calorie-restricted diet that you need. Interestingly, in the yolks, almost all the nutrients are contained.

Eggs are nutrient-dense and very filling. Eggs can reduce

hunger later in the day and even encourage weight loss compared to processed carbohydrates such as bagels.

2. Leafy Greens

Kale, spinach, collards, Swiss chards, and a few others are among the leafy greens.

They have several properties, such as being low in calories and carbohydrates and filled with fiber, making them perfect for a weight loss diet.

Eating leafy greens, without raising the calories, is a perfect way to increase the number of your meals. Numerous studies indicate that low energy intensity meals and diets help individuals consume fewer calories overall.

Leafy greens are also highly nutritious and very high in many vitamins, antioxidants, and minerals, including calcium, which in some studies has been shown to help burn fat.

Leafy greens are an impressive addition to the diet for weight loss. They are not only low in calories but also high in nutrition, which helps to keep you full.

3. The Salmon

Fatty fish such as salmon are extremely nutritious and very satisfying, keeping you full with relatively few calories for several hours.

High-quality protein, healthy fats, and various essential nutrients are filled with salmon.

A large amount of iodine can also be provided by fish and seafood in general.

For proper thyroid function, this nutrient is needed, which is necessary to keep your metabolism working optimally.

Studies indicate that a large number of individuals do not meet their iodine requirements.

Salmon is also filled with omega-3 fatty acids, which have been shown to help alleviate inflammation and play a significant role in obesity and metabolic diseases.

Often outstanding are mackerel, salmon, sardines, herring, and other types of fatty fish.

Salmon is rich in fatty acids, protein, and omega-3, making it a good option for a balanced diet for weight loss.

4. Vegetables Cruciferous

Broccoli, cauliflower, cabbage, and Brussels sprouts are among the cruciferous vegetables.

They're rich in fiber and seem to be extremely filling, like most vegetables.

What's more, in general, these kinds of veggies contain decent quantities of protein.

Unlike other vegetables, they are not nearly as rich in protein as animal foods or legumes, but still rich.

If you need to lose weight, a combination of protein, fiber, and low energy density makes cruciferous vegetables the ideal food to be included in your meals.

They're also extremely nutritious and contain substances that fight cancer.

Cruciferous vegetables are low in calories but are rich in nutrients and nutrition. Adding them to your diet is not only an outstanding technique for weight loss; it can also boost your overall health.

5. Chicken Breast and Lean Beef

Meat has been demonized unfairly.

Despite a lack of good evidence to back up these negative arguments, it has been blamed for numerous health concerns.

Studies show that unprocessed red meat does not increase the risk of heart disease or diabetes, while processed meat is unhealthy.

Red meat only has a very small association with cancer in males and no association at all in females, according to two major review studies.

The fact is since it is high in protein, meat is a weight-loss-friendly product.

Protein is by far the most nutritious food, and you can burn up to 80-100 more calories a day by eating a high-protein diet.

Studies have shown that raising your protein intake to 25-percent of daily calories will minimize cravings by 60 percent, halve your appetite for late-night snacking, and induce approximately one pound (0.45 kg) of weight loss per week.

Feel free to eat fatty meat if you're on a low-carb diet. However, if you're on a low- to a high-carbohydrate diet, it might be more fitting to choose lean meats.

An effective way to improve your consumption of protein is to eat unprocessed lean meat. It might make it easier for you to lose extra weight by replacing some of the carbohydrates or weight in your diet with protein.

6. The Boiled Potatoes

For some reason, white potatoes seem to have fallen out of favor.

However, they have several properties, both for weight loss and optimal health, that make them a perfect food.

They have an extremely varied variety of nutrients, a bit of almost everything you need.

There have been accounts of people living on nothing but potatoes alone for long periods, too.

They are extremely rich in potassium, a nutrient that is not enough for most people to get, and that plays a major role in lowering blood pressure.

The highest of all foods measured on a scale called the Satiety Index, which measures the filling of different foods, was reached by white, boiled potatoes.

What this means is that you would naturally feel full and consume less other foods by eating white, boiled potatoes.

They can shape high quantities of resistant starch, a fiber-like material that has been shown to have different health benefits, including weight loss if you allow potatoes to cool for a while after boiling.

Often outstanding are sweet potatoes, turnips, and other root vegetables.

Boiled potatoes are among the foods with the most filling. They are particularly effective at decreasing your appetite, potentially suppressing later in the day your food intake.

7. The Tuna

Another low-calorie, high-protein food is called Tuna.

They're lean fish, meaning they're low in fat.

Among bodybuilders and fitness models on a cut, Tuna is popular as it is a great way to raise protein intake while retaining low total calories and fat.

Be sure to pick tuna canned in water, not oil, if you're trying to emphasize protein intake.

Tuna is an outstanding, lean source of protein of high quality. A successful weight loss technique on a calorie-restricted diet is replacing other macronutrients, such as carbs or fat, with protein.

8. Legumes and Beans

For weight loss, some beans and other legumes may be helpful.

This involves lentils, kidney beans, black beans, and several others.

These foods, which are two nutrients that have been shown to contribute to satiety, appear to be high in protein and fiber.

They seem to produce a certain resistant starch as well.

The biggest concern is that a lot of individuals have difficulty tolerating legumes. It's important to train them properly for this purpose.

A healthy addition to the weight loss diet is beans and legumes. They are also rich in protein and fiber, leading to feelings of fullness and a lower intake of calories.

9. Soups

As described above, low energy-density meals and diets tend to make people consume fewer calories.

Those containing plenty of water, such as vegetables and fruits, are most foods with a low energy density.

But you can only add water to your food as well, to make a soup.

Some studies have shown that eating the same food has turned into a soup rather than solid food, making people feel more relaxed and consuming slightly fewer calories.

Just make sure not to add too much fat, such as cream or coconut milk, to your soup, as this may increase its calorie content significantly.

Soups may be an efficient part of a diet for weight loss. Their elevated water content makes them very complete. Try to avoid creamy or sticky soups, however.

10. Cottage Cheese

Items from dairies appear to be high in protein.

One of the best ones is cottage cheese, which is all protein with a few carbohydrates and little fat, calorie for calorie.

A perfect way to improve the consumption of protein is to eat cottage cheese. It's also very rewarding, with a relatively low number of calories to make you feel whole.

Often, dairy products are rich in calcium, which can help burn fat.

Greek yogurt and Skyr are other low-fat, high-protein dairy products.

One of the easiest ways to get more protein without drastically raising your calorie intake is consuming lean dairy products, such as cottage cheese.

11. Avocadoes

Avocados are a special fruit.

Although most fruits are high in carbohydrates, healthy fats are filled with avocados.

They are particularly high in monounsaturated oleic acid, which is the same kind of fat found in olive oil.

Avocados often contain a lot of water and fiber despite being mostly fat, making them less energy-dense than you would expect.

Moreover, they are a great addition to vegetable salads, as research indicates that their fat content can increase the absorption of carotenoid antioxidants from vegetables by 2.6 to 15 times.

Many essential nutrients, including fiber and potassium, are also present in them.

Avocados are a good example of a safe source of fat that can be used in your diet when you lose weight. Only make sure your consumption remains reasonable.

12. Vinegar with Apple Cider

Apple cider vinegar in the natural health community is extremely common.

It is also used in condiments such as dressings or vinaigrettes and is often dissolved in water and drunk by certain individuals.

Several human-based studies indicate that vinegar from apple cider may be useful for weight loss.

Simultaneously, as a high-carb meal, taking vinegar will increase feelings of fullness and make people eat 200-275 calories less for the rest of the day).

One 12-week analysis of obese individuals also found that weight loss of 2.6-3.7 pounds or 1.2-1.7 kilograms) (was caused by 15 or 30 ml of vinegar a day.

It has also been shown that vinegar decreases blood sugar spikes after meals, which in the long term can have multiple beneficial health effects).

On Amazon, you can find several types of apple cider vinegar.

It can help curb your appetite by adding apple cider vinegar to your vegetable salad, eventually leading to greater weight loss.

13. Nuts

Nuts are not as fattening as you'd expect, despite being high in fat.

It's a perfect snack with balanced quantities of protein, fiber, and healthy fats.

Research has shown that consuming nuts can enhance metabolic health and even facilitate weight loss.

Moreover, population studies have shown that individuals eating nuts appear to be healthier and leaner than those who do not.

Just make sure they don't go overboard, as the calories are still reasonably high. It might be safer to avoid them if you prefer to binge and consume large quantities of nuts.

When consumed in moderation, nuts can make a healthy addition to an efficient weight loss diet.

14. Whole Grains

In recent years, while cereal grains have gained a bad reputation, some forms are good.

This involves several whole grains that contain a good amount of protein and are filled with fiber.

Oats, brown rice, and quinoa are notable examples.

Oats are filled with beta-glucans, soluble fibers that have been shown to boost metabolic health and increase satiety.

Significant amounts of resistant starch can be present in brown and white rice, especially if cooked and then allowed to cool afterward.

Bear in mind that refined grains are not a safe option, and heavily processed snack foods that are both unhealthy and fattening are often foods with "whole grains" on the label.

You'll want to avoid grains if you're on a low-carb diet since they're high in carbohydrates.

But even if you can handle them, there is nothing wrong with eating whole grains.

If you're trying to lose weight, you should avoid refined grains. Instead, pick whole grains; they are much higher in fiber and other nutrients.

15. Chili Pepper

On a weight loss diet, consuming chili peppers can be useful.

They contain capsaicin, a compound that, in some studies, has been shown to decrease appetite and increase fat burning.

In many commercial weight loss supplements, this substance is also marketed in supplement form and is a common ingredient.

In individuals who did not eat peppers daily, one study found that consuming 1 gram of red chili pepper decreased appetite and increased fat burning.

In individuals who were accustomed to eating spicy food, however, there was no impact, suggesting that a certain degree of tolerance might build up.

Eating spicy foods containing chili peppers will temporarily reduce your appetite and even improve the burning of fat. Tolerance tends to accumulate among those who eat chili daily, however.

16. Fruits

The majority of health specialists believe that fruit is safe.

Numerous population studies have shown that individuals who consume the most fruits (and vegetables) appear to be healthier than individuals who do not.

Correlation, of course, does not equal causation, so nothing is proven by these experiments. Fruits, however, have properties that make them weight-loss-friendly.

They have a low energy density and take a while to chew, though they contain natural sugar. Plus, their fiber content helps avoid the release of sugar into your bloodstream too rapidly.

Those on a very low-carb, ketogenic diet or who have sensitivity are the only people who would want to avoid or limit fruit.

An effective and tasty addition to a weight loss diet can be an effective addition to most fruits.

While fruits contain some sugar, on a weight loss diet, you can easily include them. They are rich in nutrition, antioxidants, and nutrients, which slow down the increase in blood sugar after meals.

17. G grapefruit

Grapefruit is one fruit that needs to be highlighted. Its effects on the regulation of weight have been specifically observed.

In a 12-week study of 91 obese individuals, consuming half a fresh grapefruit before meals resulted in 3.5 pounds (1.6 kg) of weight loss.

There was also decreased insulin resistance in the grapefruit population, a metabolic abnormality implicated in multiple chronic diseases.

Therefore, about half an hour before some of your daily meals, eating half a grapefruit may help you feel more relaxed and consume fewer total calories.

Studies suggest that when eaten before meals, grapefruit can suppress appetite and decrease calorie intake. When you want to lose weight, it's worth a try.

18. Chia Seeds

Chia seeds are among the planet's most nutritious foods.

They contain 12 grams per ounce (28 grams) of carbohydrates, which is very high, but 11 grams is fiber.

This makes chia seeds a food that is low-carb-friendly and one of the world's best fiber sources.

Chia seeds can absorb up to 11-12 times their weight in water, becoming gel-like and growing in your stomach due to their high fiber content.

Although some research has shown that chia seeds can help suppress appetite, a statistically significant effect on weight loss has not been found.

However, it makes sense that chia seeds may be a useful part of your weight loss diet, considering their nutrient composition.

Chia seeds are rich in nutrition, filling you up and reducing your appetite. They may be useful on a diet for weight loss for this reason.

19. Oil from Coconut

Not all fats are equally made.

Coconut oil, or medium-chain triglycerides (MCTs), is rich in medium-length fatty acids.

It has been shown that these fatty acids improve satiety better than other fats and increase the amount of burned calories.

What's more, two studies found that coconut oil decreased quantities of belly fat, one in women and the other in men.

Of course, there are always calories in coconut oil, so putting it on top of what you are already consuming is a bad idea.

It is not about adding coconut oil to your diet, but about substituting coconut oil for some of your other cooking fats.

Studies indicate, however, that coconut oil is less satisfying than MCT oil, a substitute containing much higher medium-chain triglyceride amounts.

It is worth noting the extra virgin olive oil since this is probably one of the healthiest fats on the planet.

There are medium-chain triglycerides (MCTs) in coconut oil that can increase satiety after meals. Perhaps more effective are MCT oil supplements.

20. Yogurt Full-Fat

Yogurt is another great milk food.

Some forms of yogurt contain probiotic bacteria that can enhance your gut's work.

Getting a balanced gut will help defend against inflammation and resistance to leptin, one of obesity's key hormonal motors.

Be sure to choose yogurt with live, active cultures, because there are practically no probiotics in other forms of yogurt.

Try selecting full-fat yogurt, as well. Studies show that full-fat but not low-fat milk is associated with a decreased risk of obesity and type 2 diabetes.

Usually, low-fat yogurt is filled with sugar, so it's better to avoid it.

You will improve your digestive health with probiotic yogurt. Dream of adding it to your diet for weight loss, but make sure you avoid items with added sugar.

It is easy to find nutritious foods that should be included in a diet for weight loss.

These are mostly whole foods, such as fish, lean meat, berries, nuts, grains, vegetables, and legumes.

Several refined foods are also excellent options, such as probiotic yogurt, extra-virgin olive oil, and oatmeal.

Eating these nutritious foods, along with moderation and daily exercise, can pave the path to success and healthier life.

Chapter 14: THE GUIDE FOR HEALTHY EATING

The fast-paced contemporary world has led people to become superheroes, juggling twice as much as three jobs, yet forgetting to handle their daily food intake. If you think your body is the only weapon you have to continue to perform all the tasks you want, it is time to pay attention to its nutritional needs and satisfy them accordingly.

But starting our case from the beginning is more compelling. Millions of people who miss breakfast and have never spent the time to explore the implications of their act generally wonder why do experts consider breakfast as the most important meal of the day and how come it is still the most important meal of the day, exceeding the nutritional value of a balanced lunch or even dinner.

For millions of those who consume a nutritious breakfast, though, their path to good health lies in the first day's meal. Therefore, you need to know why eating breakfast is vital for your overall health. Your body continues to perform its functions when you are asleep, thereby consuming resources, but at a slower pace than while you are awake because your metabolism slows down to compensate for the reduced energy needs. The reduced metabolism condition is also encountered after waking up in the morning, so your body does not have enough time to return to its normal state, which can be avoided by consuming a good breakfast. That is actually why the "fasting" phase has this unique name "split." A healthy breakfast will thus end the time of calorie conservation and will allow your metabolism to rise to its normal levels. This is why you know like your energy levels have risen when you finally eat in the morning, and you are ready to begin the tasks of your day.

The food that you consume has a huge influence on your health and your quality of life.

While eating healthy can be fairly straightforward, confusion has been created by increasing common "diets" and dieting trends.

These patterns also, in fact, detract from the fundamental concepts of nutrition that are most relevant.

Based on the latest in nutrition science, this is a comprehensive beginner's guide to healthy eating.

Why do you eat nutritious food?

Analysis tends to associate extreme diseases with a bad diet

For starters, healthy eating can significantly reduce your risk of contracting heart disease and cancer, the world's leading killers.

All facets of life, from brain activity to physical efficiency, can be improved by a healthy diet. Currently, both the cells and organs are affected by food.

There is no question that a balanced diet will help you do better whether you engage in exercise or sports.

A balanced diet is important for each aspect of life, from disease risk to brain function and physical fitness.

Explained calories and Energy Balance

The value of calories has been put aside in recent years.

Although calorie counting is not always important, a key role in weight control and health is still played by total calorie intake.

You'll store them as fresh muscle or body fat if you put in more calories than you burn. You will lose weight if you eat fewer calories than you burn every day.

You must build some sort of calorie deficit if you want to lose weight.

By comparison, you need to eat more than your body burns if

you try to add weight and increase muscle mass.

Whatever the composition of your diet, calories, and energy balance is important.

Understanding Macronutrients

Carbohydrates (carbs), fats, and protein are the three macronutrients.

In relatively large quantities, these nutrients are required. They supply calories, and in your body, they have different functions.

Within a macronutrient group, here are some common foods:

- Carbs: 4 per gram of calories. Bread, pasta, and potatoes are all starchy foods. Fruit, legumes, juice, sugar, and some dairy products are also included.
- Protein: 4 per gram of calories. Meat and fish, dairy, poultry, legumes, and vegetarian alternatives, such as tofu, are major sources.
- Fats: 9 per gram of calories. The primary sources are nuts, seeds, oils, butter, cheese, fatty meat, and oily fish.

Depending on your lifestyle and priorities and your personal preferences, how much of each macronutrient you can eat.

The three key nutrients required in large quantities are macronutrients: carbohydrates, fats, and protein.

UNDERSTANDING MICRONUTRIENTS

In smaller doses, micronutrients are essential vitamins and minerals that you need.

Some of the most prevalent micronutrients that you can understand include:

Magnesium: Plays a role in over 600 cellular processes, including the production of energy, operation of the nervous system, and contraction of muscles.

Potassium: This mineral is vital for regulating blood pressure, fluid balance, and muscle and nerve function.

Iron: Iron also has many other advantages, including enhanced immune and brain function, primarily known for carrying oxygen in the blood.

Calcium: A significant bone and teeth structural factor, and also a vital mineral for your heart, muscles, and nervous system.

All vitamins: In every organ and cell in your body, vitamins, from vitamin A to K, play an important role.

All the vitamins and minerals are "important" nutrients, meaning that to survive, you must get them from the diet.

Each micronutrient's daily requirement differs between individuals. If you eat a true diet that includes plants and animals dependent on fruit, then without taking a supplement, you can get all the micronutrients your body needs.

Micronutrients are essential vitamins and minerals in your cells and organs that play key roles.

It's important to eat whole food

At least 80-90 percent of the time, you should aim to consume whole foods.

In general, the term "whole food" describes natural, unprocessed foods that contain only one ingredient.

If the food looks like it was manufactured in a factory, it may not be an entire meal.

Whole foods have a lower energy density and tend to be

nutrient-dense. This suggests that they have fewer calories and more nutrients than refined foods per serving.

Many refined foods, on the other hand, have no nutritional value and are also regarded as "empty" calories. Eating them in large quantities is linked to obesity and other illnesses.

An extremely efficient but simple strategy for improving health and losing weight is to base your diet on whole foods.

Foods for Eat

Try to base your diet on these classes of balanced foods:

Vegetables: For most meals, these can play a key role. They are low in calories and full of fiber and essential micronutrients.

Fruits: Fruits contain micronutrients and antioxidants that can help improve health as a naturally sweet treat.

Meat and fish: Meat and fish throughout nature have been the main sources of protein. In the human diet, they are a staple, although vegetarian and vegan diets have also become common.

Nuts and seeds: These are some of the best available sources of fat and contain substantial micronutrients.

Eggs: Considered one of the healthiest foods on the planet, a good balance of protein, beneficial fats, and micronutrients is filled with whole eggs (20).

Dairy: Dairy products are easy, low-cost sources of protein and calcium, such as natural yogurt and milk.

Stable starches: All starchy foods such as potatoes, quinoa, and Ezekiel bread are healthy and nutritious for those not on a low-carb diet.

Beans and legumes: These are great fiber, protein, and micronutrient sources.

Beverages: Water, along with beverages like coffee and tea, can make up the bulk of your fluid intake.

Herbs and spices: These are also very rich in nutrients and plant compounds that are beneficial.

On these balanced, whole foods and ingredients, base your diet. All the nutrients your body needs will be provided by them.

Foods that you can stop most of the time

You would automatically decrease your consumption of unhealthy foods by following the advice in this post.

No food needs to be removed permanently, but for special occasions, those items should be reduced or saved.

They include:

Sugar-based products: sugar-rich foods, especially sugary beverages, are linked to obesity and type 2 diabetes.

Trans fats: Also known as partially hydrogenated fats, trans fats, such as heart disease have been linked to serious illnesses.

Refined carbs: Overeating, obesity, and metabolic disease are linked to foods that are high in refined carbs, such as white bread.

Vegetable oils: While many people assume they are safe, vegetable oils can affect the omega 6-to-3 balance of your body, causing problems.

Low-fat products processed: Low-fat products often disguised as nutritious substitutes typically contain a lot of sugar to make them taste better.

While no food is strictly off-limits, overeating such foods can increase the risk of disease and contribute to weight gain.

WHY CONTROL OF PORTIONS IS ESSENTIAL

A crucial element in weight gain and wellbeing is calorie consumption.

You are more likely to stop eating too many calories by limiting your portions.

While whole foods are probably much more difficult to overeat than refined foods, they can still be consumed excessively.

It's especially important to control your portion size if you are overweight or trying to lose body fat.

To control portion size, there are several basic techniques.

You can use smaller plates, for instance, and take a smaller-than-average first serving, then wait 20 minutes before returning for more.

Measuring portion size with your hand is another common method. Most individuals will be limited to 1 fist-sized portion of carbohydrates, 1-2 protein palms, and 1-2 thumb-sized portions of healthy fats in an example meal.

More calorie-dense foods are good, such as cheese, nuts, and fatty meats, so make sure that when you consume them, you pay attention to portion sizes.

Be mindful of the portions and your overall intake of food or calories, especially if you are overweight or trying to lose fat.

How to tailor your diet for your goals

Next, depending on variables such as your activity levels and weight targets, determine your calorie needs.

Very clearly, you have to eat less than you burn if you want to lose weight. You can eat more calories than you lose if you want to gain weight.

Here is a calorie tracker that tells you how much you can consume, and here are five free calorie and nutrient tracking websites and applications.

If you hate calorie counting, you should simply add the rules mentioned above, such as portion size control and concentrating on whole foods.

You may need to adjust your diet to account for this if you have a certain deficiency or are at risk of developing one. For example, certain nutrients are at greater risk of losing out on vegetarians or individuals who exclude such food groups.

In general, to ensure you get enough of both the macro- and micronutrients, you can eat foods of different types and colors.

While many are debating whether low-carb or low-fat diets are better, the reality is that it depends on the individual.

Athletes and others trying to lose weight should consider increasing their protein intake, based on studies. Furthermore, for some people trying to lose weight or treat type 2 diabetes, a lower-carb diet can work wonders.

Accept your overall consumption of calories and change your diet based on your desires and objectives.

HOW TO MAINTAIN HEALTHY EATING

Here's a great law to live by: If in one, two, or three years, you can't see yourself on this diet, then it's not right for you.

People go on strict diets that they can't manage, way too often, meaning they never really develop long-term, balanced eating habits.

Some frightening weight gain figures indicate that soon after trying a weight loss diet, most individuals regain all the weight they lost.

Balance is important, as always. If you have a particular illness or dietary necessity, there is no need for food to forever be off-limits. You can potentially increase cravings and decrease long-term success by fully removing those foods.

Basing 90% of your diet on whole foods and consuming smaller portions would allow you to periodically enjoy treats but still achieve outstanding health.

This is a much better solution than doing the reverse and consuming, as many people do, 90% processed food and just 10% natural food.

For the long term, build a balanced diet that you can enjoy and stick with. Save them for an occasional treat if you want unhealthy foods.

Think of these supplements

Supplements are intended to be used in addition to a balanced diet, as the name implies.

It can help you reverse deficiencies and fulfill all your daily needs by having plenty of nutrient-dense foods in your diet.

However, in some cases, a few well-researched supplements are beneficial.

Vitamin D, which is naturally obtained from sunlight and foods such as oily fish, is one case. Some individuals have low levels or are deficient.

If you do not get enough of them from your diet, supplements such as magnesium, zinc, and omega-3s can offer additional advantages.

To boost athletic results, other supplements may be used. All have plenty of evidence supporting their use, including creatine, whey protein, and beta-alanine.

Your diet will be full of nutrient-dense foods and no need for supplements in a perfect world. In the real world, though, this is not always feasible.

Additional supplements will help to take your wellbeing a step further if you are already making a daily effort to boost your diet.

Having most of your nutrients from whole foods is best. Nevertheless, certain supplements can also be helpful.

Combine other healthy practices with good nutrition

Nutrition, for good health, is not the only thing that matters.

You will get an even bigger health boost by adopting a balanced diet and exercising.

Having a good sleep is also important. Research demonstrates that sleep is just as important for disease risk and weight control as a diet.

Also essential are hydration and water intake. Drink the entire day when you're thirsty and stay well hydrated.

Try to alleviate tension, eventually. Many health conditions are related to long-term stress.

Optimal health goes far deeper than nutrition alone. It is also important to practice, get good sleep, and reduce stress.

The methods outlined above will improve your diet significantly.

They will also improve your fitness, lower the risk of your infection, and help you lose weight.

HOW TO DEFEAT FOOD ADDICTION

The effects on the brain of such foods make it impossible for certain individuals to stop them.

Food addiction acts similarly to other addictions, which

explains why, no matter how hard they try, some people can't control themselves around those foods.

They can find themselves consuming large quantities of unhealthy foods frequently, despite not wanting to, knowing that doing so may cause harm.

This book looks at food addiction and offers tips for overcoming it.

WHAT IS AN ADDICTION TO FOOD?

Food addiction is a fast food addiction that is similar to opioid addiction.

It's a relatively new and controversial concept, and there is a shortage of high-quality data about its prevalence.

Food addiction, including binge eating disorder, bulimia, compulsive overeating, and other feeding and eating disorders, is similar to other disorders.

A particularly debated term is food addiction, although most researchers say that it exists. Similarly to opioid abuse, it works.

Impact on the brain

The same regions of the brain as opioid addiction are concerned with food addiction. It also includes the same neurotransmitters, and many of the signs are similar.

Processed junk meals have a strong effect on the brain's reward centers. Brain neurotransmitters such as dopamine (3) induce these results.

Typical unhealthy foods such as candy, sugary soda, and high-fat fried foods are among the most harmful foods.

Food addiction is not induced by a lack of willpower but is

thought to be triggered by a signal from dopamine that influences the brain's biochemistry.

It is believed that food addiction includes the same neurotransmitters and areas of the brain as opioid addiction.

Eight food addiction signs

A blood test to detect food addiction does not exist. It's focused on behavioral signs, as in other addictions.

Here are eight common symptoms:

1. Despite feeling full and having just finished a healthy meal, daily cravings for some foods
2. Eating the desired meal and always eating much more than expected
3. Eating the desired meal and always eating to the point of feeling overstuffed
4. After eating specific foods, they sometimes feel guilty, and consume them again shortly after.
5. Often make excuses for why it is a good idea to respond to a food craving
6. Trying to avoid eating certain foods frequently, but unsuccessfully, or setting rules for eating them is permitted, such as at cheat meals or on certain days,
7. The intake of unhealthy foods is also concealed from others.
8. Also, recognizing that they cause physical damage or weight gain, they feel powerless to regulate the intake of unhealthy foods.

It may mean that there is a deeper problem if more than four or five of the symptoms on this list apply. If there are six or more, so it's probably a food addiction.

Craving and binging on unhealthy foods without being hungry and an inability to fight the temptation to consume these foods are the main signs of food addiction.

It is a serious issue

Although the word addiction is often tossed around loosely, a severe illness that usually needs medication to cure is getting a genuine addiction.

The food addiction-related signs and cognitive processes are close to those of substance abuse. It's just a different drug, and there could be less serious social ramifications.

Physical damage can be caused by food abuse and contribute to chronic health problems such as obesity and type 2 diabetes.

Furthermore, it can adversely affect the self-esteem and self-image of a person, making them dissatisfied with their body.

Food addiction can take an emotional toll, as with other addictions, and increase a person's risk of premature death.

The risk of obesity and type 2 diabetes is increased by food addiction. Also, excessive weight can affect the self-esteem of an individual.

How to learn if the sacrifice is worth avoiding junk food

It can seem difficult to stop junk food altogether. They're everywhere and a big part of popular society.

In certain situations, however, it can become important to abstain from such trigger foods.

When the firm decision to never consume these foods again is made, it will become easier to avoid them as they are removed by the desire to justify eating or not to eat them. Cravings can disappear or dramatically decrease, as well.

To think about the decision, consider writing a list of pros and cons.

• Pros. This could include weight loss, living longer, getting more energy, and every day feeling better.

• Cons. These could include the lack of family ice cream, no cookies during the holiday season, and the need to justify food choices.

No matter how odd or vain it may seem, write all down. Compare the two lists then and ask if it's worth it.

If a resounding "yes" is the answer, be sure it is the right decision.

Often, bear in mind that it can also quickly overcome many social dilemmas that might arise in the con list.

An individual should be confident that removing such foods is the correct thing to overcome food addiction. If there's doubt, writing down the pros and cons will help make a choice.

First steps towards overcoming food addiction

A few items can help plan for the abandonment of junk foods and promote the transition:

Cause foods. Write down a list of the foods triggering cravings and/or binges. These are the cause of food for complete avoidance.

Fast food locations. Make a list of locations for fast food that serve nutritious foods and acknowledge their healthier choices. When hungry and not in the mood to cook, this can avoid a relapse.

About what to eat. Think of what foods to consume, ideally nutritious foods that are frequently enjoyed and already consumed.

Pros and cons. • Try having many pro-and-con list copies. Keep a copy in your bathroom, purse or wallet, and glove box.

Moreover, don't go on a diet. For at least 1–3 months, put weight loss on hold.

It is difficult enough to resolve food addiction. It is possible that adding hunger and constraints to the mix would make things harder.

Set a date shortly, such as the coming weekend, after taking these preparatory steps, from which point the addictive trigger foods will not be touched again.

It's important to prepare to conquer food addiction. Create a list of trigger foods and know instead what will be consumed.

Try seeking assistance

Most addicted individuals try to stop several times before succeeding in the long run.

Although it is possible without assistance to conquer addiction, even though it takes many attempts, it can also help seek support.

To conquer the addiction, several health practitioners and support groups will help.

It can include one-on-one counseling to find a counselor or therapist who has experience coping with food addiction, but there are also many community group options available.

That includes 12-step services such as Overeaters Anonymous (OA), Food Addicts Anonymous (FAA), GreySheeters Anonymous (GSA), and Food Addicts in Recovery Anonymous (FA).

These groups meet regularly and can provide the help required to overcome addiction, some even through video chat.

Consider looking for food abuse support. Try support groups such as Overeaters Anonymous or book an appointment with a specialist food addiction psychologist or therapist.

Food addiction is an issue that never fixes on its own. Unless a deliberate effort is taken to deal with it, it will possibly intensify over time.

Listing the pros and cons of stopping trigger foods, seeking healthier food alternatives, and setting a defined date to begin the path towards wellness are the first steps to overcoming the addiction.

Try finding assistance from a free support network or health provider. Always bear in mind that you are not alone.

8 COMMON FOOD ADDICTION SYMPTOMS

Although food addiction is not described in the Mental Disorders Diagnostic and Statistical Manual (DSM-5), it usually includes binge eating habits, cravings, and a lack of food control.

Although often anyone who gets a craving or overeats will certainly not meet the condition definition, there are at least eight typical symptoms.

Here are eight signs and symptoms of food addiction that are typical.

1. Gaining cravings despite feeling full

Even after consuming a satisfying, healthy meal, it's not normal to get cravings.

Some people may crave ice cream for dessert after eating dinner with steak, potatoes, and veggies.

Cravings and starvation are not the same things.

A craving happens when, despite having already eaten or been full, you feel a desire to consume something.

This is very normal and doesn't necessarily suggest that anyone is addicted to food. The majority of individuals get cravings.

However, if cravings arise regularly, and it becomes difficult to satisfy or ignore them, they may indicate something else.

These cravings are not about the need for energy or nutrients; the brain calls for something that stimulates dopamine, a brain chemical that plays a part in how humans perceive pleasure.

Cravings are very popular. Although craving alone does not mean food addiction, it can indicate a problem if you often get cravings, and it is hard to ignore or satisfy them.

2. Eating a lot more than expected

There is no such thing as a bite of chocolate or a single slice of cake for certain people. One bite turns into 20, and half a cake turns into one slice of cake.

With the addition of any sort, this all-or-nothing approach is popular. There's no such thing as moderation; it's just not working.

Saying to consume fast food in moderation to food addiction is almost like asking someone with alcoholism to drink beer in moderation. It just isn't true.

Someone with a food addiction might consume much more than expected while giving in to a craving.

3. Eating up until you feel overly bloated

When giving in to compulsion, before the urge is fulfilled, someone with food addiction can not stop eating. They may then realize they have eaten so much that they feel bloated in their stomach.

Eating until you feel overly bloated can be known as binge eating, either regularly or all the time.

4. Feeling guilty later, but soon do it again

Trying to exercise control over excessive food intake and then giving in to a craving can lead to feelings of guilt.

A person may feel like they are doing something wrong or even cheating themselves.

An individual with food addiction will repeat the pattern despite these unpleasant feelings.

Feelings of shame are common after a time of binge eating.

5. Making up excuses

Especially in regards to addiction, the brain can be a strange thing. It may lead anyone to create rules for themselves by trying to stay away from trigger foods. But, it may be hard to obey these laws.

Someone with food addiction can find ways to reason around the rules when faced with craving and give in to the craving.

This line of thought may mimic that of a person who is trying to quit smoking. The person may think that they are not a smoker if they don't buy a pack of cigarettes themselves. Nonetheless, they could smoke a friend's pack of cigarettes.

It can be normal with food addiction to set rules about eating habits and then make excuses about why it's appropriate to follow them.

6. Repeated delays in laying down rules

They also attempt to set rules for themselves while individuals are struggling with self-control.

Examples include only sleeping in on the weekends, always doing homework right after school, never drinking coffee in the afternoon after a certain time. These laws almost always fail for most individuals, and laws about eating are no exception.

For example, one cheats meal or cheat day every week and

consuming only fast food at parties, birthdays, or holidays are included.

Many individuals have at least some history of failing to create guidelines on their intake of food.

7. Hiding eating from others

Individuals with a history of rule-setting and frequent failures also begin to mask their junk food intake from others.

When no one else is home, alone in the car, or late at night after everyone else has gone to bed, they may choose to eat alone.

Among individuals who feel unable to regulate their eating, hiding food intake is fairly normal.

8. Unable to stop despite physical issues

Whatever foods you want to eat will affect your health significantly.

Junk food can lead to weight gain, acne, bad breath, tiredness, poor dental health, and other common problems in the short term.

Obesity, type 2 diabetes, heart disease, Alzheimer's, dementia, and even certain kinds of cancer can lead to a lifetime of junk food consumption.

One who has all of these concerns linked to their ingestion of unhealthy foods but is unwilling to alter their behaviors would require assistance.

For managing eating disorders, a treatment plan developed by trained practitioners is usually recommended.

It can be impossible to avoid, even when unhealthy eating habits cause physical problems.

The DSM-5 is a guide that is used to evaluate mental illnesses by health professionals.

Many of the signs above are included in the criterion for drug dependency. They suit in with medical addiction concepts. The DSM-5 has not, however, laid down guidelines for food addiction.

If you have consistently tried to avoid eating or cut down on your junk food intake but can't, it may be a food addiction sign.

CONCLUSION

If you think your body is the only weapon you have to continue to perform all the tasks you want, it is time to pay attention to its nutritional needs and satisfy them accordingly.

The fast-paced contemporary world has led people to become superheroes, juggling twice as much as three jobs, yet forgetting to handle their daily food intake.

Many individuals have indicated that after going through hypnosis for weight loss services because they feel fuller longer and quicker after a small meal, they don't eat as much as before.

You've already noticed that eating a nutritious breakfast will save you from cravings later in the day and will potentially help you shed the extra weight that you've been carrying around for some time now. But, as time has lately been considered a luxury, not many people have during the day. Particularly during a busy weekday morning, it is now a forgotten nutritional habit to start the day off by eating a healthy breakfast.

Goal-setting methods will be taught, and you will learn precisely what to do, how to accomplish your goals, and how to measure success. A positive feedback loop will produce results during your hypnosis weight loss plan and motivate you to stay on track and meet the weight loss goals you set for yourself.

The hypnosis of weight loss is, therefore, real and is now helping individuals from all walks of life achieve their weight loss goals and give them control of their lives by giving them a safe and easy way to achieve their desired level of health.

RAPID WEIGHT LOSS HYPNOSIS

INTRODUCTION

Weight loss goes down to the idea of calories in, calories out: Drink less than you eat, and you're going to lose weight. And while water weight can be easily lost on a low-carb diet, I will not be advocating for it. The food itself would make you believe that this style of eating works — when you get back what you lost as soon as you eat carbs again. When you want results that last longer than a week, it can feel incredibly dispiriting.

Based on my nutrition counselling experience, most of us prefer to snack foods that aren't nutrient-dense but are high in calories. Of starters, avoiding sugary drinks is also the best way to lose weight faster. Many big culprits, including chips, cereals, crackers, and cookies, also come in processed grains.

I would always encourage you to be aware of the stuff you eat that you don't want for yourself when you're trying to boost weight loss. Think of food pushers at work or baby leftovers. Noticing where the extra calories come from is just another step in making healthier short- and long-term decisions.

When weight loss is explicitly discussed in its serious exposition, we all admit and encourage this normal and general knowledge as the basic way to achieve weight loss which is the apt involvement of medical expertise: private trainers, health instructors, mental health personnel, nutritionists, dietitians, and medical doctors. Will catch you aghast to reveal to you that we haven't thought of an unexplored idea which is a hypnotist.

The option to use hypnosis as another interesting route to make the weight loss effective and workable is, in turn, the lane on which many thread. Optimistically, the so-called general ideology and the way out of weight loss are undoubtedly not working as it is said to be. People have implemented methods based on methods, yet many tend to live in ample disappointment based on non-actualizing prescribed workouts and principles.

In the heart of many, there have been a lot of confusions, claims and incoherencies against a limpid perception of what hypnosis means. Many have resolved to say; it's just about manipulating one 's mind and making the other do things against one's will. These and more are the miss-appropriated knowledge about hypnosis nurtured by many.

You may not be conscious of the external experiences around you during hypnosis. Before entering gross sleep, it is in the form of a deep state of rest and a semi-medium realm. It is the state when, as in a dose, you seem to be partially cut off from the relation of your immediate world, but still have a sense of very minute knowledge of what's happening around you.

A state like this opens you up and gives you over to possible improvements, which can result in the effect of weight loss through hypnosis. Hypnosis varies from most other treatments in the sense that it focuses its behaviors on one's subconscious state of mind, thereby influencing one's negative self-talk, habits, food choices, self-esteem, memory and emotional stability. Before that, hardly do we have any other techniques that discuss and influence the real problems to its roots as hypnosis does.

When it comes to losing weight: you are aware of the regular go-to professionals: doctors, dietitians and nutritionists, personal trainers, and mental health coaches. Yet there might be one that you haven't even heard yet: a hypnotist.
Using hypnosis turns out to be another path people go down in the name of weight loss. And usually, it's done after all the other last-ditch attempts (I see you, fad diets and juice cleanses) are being tried and failed, says Greg Gurniak, an Ontario-based accredited clinical and medical hypnotist.
But it's not about someone else manipulating your mind when you're asleep and making you do crazy stuff. "Mind control and lack of power — aka doing it against your will — are the biggest myths regarding hypnosis," says Kimberly Friedmutter,

hypnotherapist and author of Subconscious Power: Using Your Inner Mind to Create the Life Yo
u've always desired. "Due to the way the entertainment industry depicts hypnotists, people are pleased to see that I don't wear a black robe and swing a watch from a chain." Even when you undergo hypnosis, you are not unconscious — it's more of a deep state of relaxation, Friedmutter says. "It's just the normal, floaty feeling you get before you sleep, or the dreamy feeling you get when you wake up in the morning before you're completely conscious of where you're and what's around you."

What is the relationship between Hypnosis and weight-loss?

Hypnosis is something that we like to find as a kind of fun, but have you ever thought of weight-loss Hypnosis? It is trying to use Hypnosis to cope with a situation as extreme as weight issues, so maybe it's not as crazy as it seems. Weight-loss Hypnosis is an enticing concept-it gives people a fairly easy way out of their weight issue by preventing their appetite for food at the source.

One weight-loss dilemma by Hypnosis is the same issue that affects other approaches to weight-reduction.

There are plenty scams out there, and the people behind them do not hesitate to try to take your money for a product that does nothing at all. Hypnosis does have the same problem. You may be able to trust some statements regarding weight-loss therapy for Hypnosis; however, there are just as many who have loads of lies.

If weight-loss treatment hypnosis declares it can help you lose some insane number of pounds in a few weeks or similar exaggerations, it is pretty safe to bet it's a scam. If you find claims that say that Hypnosis can alter the way the mind works to avoid eating, they are likely to be deceiving.

As you sleep or wake up from sleep, your mind goes through the various stages of brainwave operation. Bata's where you're now if you don't dream, that's it. The waves are high. There is Alpha just under that knowledge. The waves are slower and awake but in a modified state of consciousness. Have you ever driven your car, and you're just thinking about your questioning where you were at the exit? Yeah, when driving, you've got your mind attached to the Alpha zone. When under Hypnosis, this is the same thing the brain does. Keep in mind when driving the car that you kept in control, that you hit nothing, that's the same with Hypnosis. Theta comes under the Alphah; you don't sleep but go to sleep. And you're unconscious, known as the Delta. When you get up, you are going in reverse through those brainwave states.

Now that we understand the workings of our minds let's start talking about Hypnosis. Hypnosis is the workaround within the conscious mind of the vital dimension and the establishment of embracing discerning thoughts. Notice that the definition does not say something about relaxing or giving up control? Hypnosis is more of a natural condition.

Chapter 1: HISTORY OF HYPNOSIS

Hypnosis has existed as a solution to the unconscious and encouraging the unconscious to help the subconscious accomplish the necessary changes and advantages, as long as we choose to change behavior. Such actions wouldn't have been considered hypnosis, but hadn't been hypnotic until Braid did 1842.

A treatment was discussed in the Ebers Papyrus in which the physician placed his hands on the patient's head and declared superhuman healing powers offered with original remedial utterances that were recommended to the patients, and that led to treatments.

The famous figure in the history of Hypnosis in the 18th century was Dr. Frantz Anton Mesmer (1734-1815), an Austrian physician who used magnets and metal frames to carry out "passes" over the client to remove "obstructions" (causes of disease) in the body's magnetic forces and induce a trance-like state. In 1784, Dr. Mesmer's trainee, the Marquis de Puysegur, discovered how to lead a patient into a deep hypnotic trance state called "somnambulism," using relaxation techniques. The word "somnambulism" is still commonly used today by hypnotherapists in comparison to a deep hypnotic state of trance and sleep-walking.

This technique was used by French physicians, consisting of Dr. Recamier, who conducted the first recorded procedure without anesthesia in 1821 for several years following. The Marquis de Puysegur described three principal functions of this state of deep hypnotic trance or somnambulism.

In 1841, a Scottish optometrist, Dr. James Braid (1775-1860), discovered through an accident that a private fixation on an object might easily enter a hypnotic trance state without Dr. Mesmer 's approval of the mesmeric effect. He published his observations, denied the work of Mesmer, and mistakenly named his theory "hypnotherapy" based on the Greek word "Hypnos," which means "sleep." It was a wrong option because Hypnosis is not sleeping; however, the term has stayed, and mesmerism has become hypnotherapy.

He formulated the following ideas during Braid's research study of Hypnosis, the majority of which still stand today:

1) This is a professional hand, there is no substantial chance of hypnotic therapy, and there is no pain or discomfort either.
2) To better understand some theoretical concepts relating to Hypnosis, an excellent research study would be required.
3) Hypnosis is one powerful tool that must be confined entirely to qualified experts.
4) While hypnotism was capable of curing various diseases for which no established care had been given, it was not, however, a panacea and was merely a therapeutic technique that could be used in combination with other medical knowledge, medications, medicines, etc., to treat the client appropriately.

However, in his early work Sigmund Freud (1856-1939), the dad of psychoanalysis, using Hypnosis, was disillusioned by the theory. There's an assumption he didn't have the anesthetic dedication and wasn't an excellent hypnotist. About 1883-1887, he was fascinated with Hypnosis and studied for a while, and Freud spent some time with Charcot in 1885 and was amazed. He also translated De la Suggestion, by German Bernheim.

In Vienna, Freud and his buddy Joseph Breuer successfully used Hypnosis in psychotherapy and 1895, and they developed their typical 'Studies in Hysteria' that Freud had checked out Nancy in 1889, and this experience had convinced him of the 'important psychological mechanisms that remain concealed from male consciousness.' On this, Freud wrote, 'I was humble enough not to attribute the incident to my own compelling personal attraction, and I felt I had now understood the essence of the mystical factor behind hypnotism that was at work.'

The pioneer to modern-day Hypnosis and self-advancement was Dr. Emile Coué (1857-1926), who at the end of the 19th century believed in self-suggestion and the role of the hypnotherapist as a facilitator of transformation and healing, using the client's complete participation in the process of Hypnosis. By 1887 Coué established the theory of self-suggestion, which is perhaps the very first ego-strengthening (a cornerstone of traditional occult and shamanic practices) that the modern scientific community had used. He thought about the importance of imagination in directing a person's will and conducted experiments to determine how individuals' suggestions affected their behavior.

His well-known statement of self-help: "Day by day in every way I am changing and progressing," is still used in most self-improvement therapies.

1. Coue's Laws of Suggestion: The Law of Concentrated Attention-" If attention is turned to an idea over and over again, it appears to recognize itself spontaneously.
2. The Law of Reverse Action-" The more you try to do something and the less chance you have of succeeding.
3. The Dominant Effect Theory-" A stronger emotion appears to take the place of a weaker one.

Coue believed he could not cure people by himself but only encouraged their self-healing, so he recognized the importance of the subject's participation in Hypnosis, a precursor to the assumption that 'there is no such thing as hypnosis, just self-hypnosis.' Probably his most famous theory was that imagination is always more powerful than will. For example, if you ask anyone on the floor to walk along with a wood slab, they will do it without wobbling in general.

Hypnosis categories

For decades, Hypnosis has been used as a tool for shocking, impressing, and helping to heal and treat. With or without any method, the principles of Hypnosis remain the same; however, there are different ways to achieve this. Usually, the form of anesthesia used relies on the desired outcome.

Hypnotherapeutic

The use of Hypnosis in some form is known as hypnotherapy to facilitate recovery or successful development. Equally, hypnotherapy can be used to regulate pain stimuli, and Hypnosis has been used to perform surgery on patients who are completely aware of it. If not for the use of anesthesia, they would be in obvious pain.

Hypnosis may be used to help women. Hypnotherapy may be highly effective for psychological disorders, such as anxiety. Fears, attachments, and all manner of false beliefs can be reprogrammed selectively, and negative emotions controlled. Hypnosis, as used in hypnotherapy, may also have practical effects, the most common being to avoid pain by allowing surgical operations to be done without the anesthetic-related damage and risks.

Hypnotherapy also uses Hypnosis of intense lightness, not the deep coma state has seen in the conventional form.

The main point of the hypnotherapy is that the patient should stay focused on the medication and understand the words that the therapist says.

Ericksonian Hypnotization

This method of Hypnosis has many names, concealed Hypnosis, hidden Hypnosis, Hypnosis of the black ops, instant Hypnosis, Hypnosis of conversations. This approach uses frequent conversation and encourages hypnotic induction without the subject being aware that it is happening.

Hypnotherapist Dr. Milton H. Erickson began Ericksonian Hypnosis or conversational Hypnosis. After being ill with polio Erickson mastered the use of words, holding him in bed for many years. During this time, he perfected ways of using traditional conversation to cause hypnotic states without understanding the subject.

This method of Hypnosis can be used on those who are uncertain about hypnotherapy or more conventional Hypnosis, and those who are more skeptical are said to be more effective on those.

This technique can be used on those wary of Hypnosis or unaware of being hypnotized. In normal speech, the use of hypnotic language and Hypnosis techniques can trigger trance quickly.

This technique of Hypnosis was initially established as a strategy for hypnotherapy, but it has ended up being used more in everyday life by everyday people. The program helps the client to take full control of their lives and use these strategies to assist them in many everyday scenarios. The procedure is relatively straightforward, but mastering the system will take time.

• Hypnosis/Self-hypnosis

It is comparable with Hypnosis and self-hypnosis. The hypnotherapist is merely the auto that assists the subject in a trance; nevertheless, the subject processes the knowledge, but the result is the same.

Self-hypnosis can be immensely used for hypnotherapy and is effective in resolving mental disorders, anxiety, tension, and dependencies. Usually, it is used only to facilitate a state of deep relaxation.

NLP Hypnosis

The NLP technique is still commonly used; however, it is now more commonly used as a self-help method to support and encourage feelings of well-being. This technique has an increasingly growing popularity and is used by customer consultants, support specialists, life coaches, and self-help courses.

NLP hypnosis is used to resolve psychological or behavioral issues, or simply to enhance one's sense of well-being. This is a great tool to encourage and build faith in oneself.

Modern Hypnosis

The classic design of anesthesia is conventional Hypnosis and has been around for a long time. This is the version performed by a psychiatrist who puts the subject into a deep hypnotic trance and then directs it using ideas and commands. This approach is used by Stage hypnotism.

Throughout the years, the modern form of Hypnosis has been much maligned and ridiculed, often unjustified, but sadly, some of the criticism is right. The real traditional hypnosis technique has been weakened by the use of artificial Hypnosis using plants and performers. It is a reliable and essential tool, which can be very useful when applied appropriately.

Important of Hypnosis For Women

Hypnosis can help individuals handle:

- Fears.
- Post-op surgery bleeding and pain.
- Labour and childbirth.
- Dental treatment recovery.
- Migraine headaches.
- Chemotherapy nausea,/vomiting.
- Asthma.
- Weak body immune systems.
- High blood pressure.
- Irritable Bowel Syndrome discomfort.
- Anxiety disorders, stress.
- Skin illness.

- Negative behaviors like eating conditions, smoking cigarettes, drug abuse, bedwetting.
- Atopic and psoriasis dermatitis.

Hypnosis is used to help a person relax, helping them to end up being much more relaxed and confident. During a consultation with hypnotherapy, a person with chronic pain can achieve a whole new degree of relaxation. A brand-new state of relaxation will assist them in fighting anxiety, reduce issues at work and home, and generally help them cope better with the pain.

In some people, the Hypnosis works even better than for others. The patient has to be willing to work for the treatment. It is equally important to the success of hypnotherapy that the patient is prepared to handle the suggestions coming out of the session.

There are options for Hypnosis. A consultation with an experienced hypnotherapist will assist you in finding the approach that is best for you.

Let's think about what self-hypnosis is before we join what it can and can't do for us. If you've ever been to a hypnotherapist, you may have been told that self-hypnosis is all Hypnosis. All this means is that without your consent or participation, no one will get you into a trance.

Absolutely nothing could be further from the truth. Hypnosis is a natural state of mind in which we all participate, many times a day. You live in a hypnotic state at any time. Your mind is so concentrated that you are not aware of what's going on around you. Whether it's seeing TELEVISION or reading or playing, we remain in a state of Hypnosis whenever we slip out of today and dive into our minds and focus our attention.

Naturally, when we talk about self-hypnosis in a therapeutic context, we don't think about such experiences. We are talking about a systematic process in which we take our attention away from our present environments and place ourselves in a different state of mind for a particular reason.

And how are we doing the self-hypnosis?

There are as many ways to do self-hypnosis as there are individuals, but I will explain a reliable yet basic approach that anyone can do for this book.

The very first thing you want to do is to find a quiet place where you won't be disturbed. Treat yourself to a nice half-hour. Turn down the phone and ask the children to be quiet and have fun at this time. Nevertheless, in an emergency, realize that you will be immediately activated and return to normal walking without difficulty.

Get relaxed, be it sitting down or lying down. You can have soft music in the background if you like. Many meditative music recordings are suitable for self-hypnosis. Some people use music to relax more deeply with them.

Now concentrate on breathing. Feel the breath going in and out of the nose. Feel the air entering your body. See, this fluctuates in your tummy. The breathing exercise is also followed by the concept of "Calming in relaxation and calmness and calming our stress and anxiety."

You may also use relaxation to put you back into a state of deep peace and tranquility. Picture the muscles around your head, start relaxing, and getting limp. Then take the feeling to your head 's peak. Feel all the muscles inside your back, head and face, let go and unwind. Using this technique to go all the way down your whole body, relax and unwind.

Using terms like "deeper and deeper into relaxation," "moving down," "calm, peaceful relaxation," etc. in your mind as you breathe and feel all the stress that goes out of your muscles.

Reverse counting is another good way to get further into relaxation. "decreasing 10, ... 9 half as confident as before, ... 8 constantly falling ... and so on."

Everyone's having a distinct experience going into Hypnosis. Pay attention to the senses, and see how Hypnosis you'll feel. A lot of people would wonder at this moment, "What is the difference between self-hypnosis and meditation?"

Meditation is a practice where you clear your mind. Hypnosis is comparable because you can unwind and see your breathing, but the resemblances end here. Hypnosis has a specific purpose behind it because instead of being translucent, the mind is especially active, but differently than the normal state of consciousness.

You are going with the intention to go through Hypnosis. If the reason you use Hypnosis is for relief from stress, for example, you may carry the purpose of 'I'm calm and comfortable all day long.

Imagination plays a major part in Hypnosis. Perceiving or anticipating the outcome that you want helps to integrate the idea into your subconscious mind. If the idea stays in your subconscious mind, it ends up being a part of your everyday life.

When you think about anything enough, or visualize it, your subconscious mind will have it in your life. When you go into self-hypnosis with a particular purpose in mind and repeat the goal, it ends up being a part of you.

When you are in Hypnosis, and you have a superior, you will find that this is a part of your mind that is still in charge. It is the part of your account that is going to repeat the aim. This will also, at the agreed-upon time, get you out of the Hypnosis.

Coming out of the state of Hypnosis to yourself, "I'm going to count from one to five now, and I'm going to open my eyes on the count of five and return to normal awakening." "One, turning up slowly ..., 2, feeling refreshed and restful and happy ..., three, feeling my body back in the bed ..., 4, recalling every advantageous thing I've said to my subconscious mind today ..., five, all the way up, eyes open."

Bear in mind that if you are giving yourself a suggestion to repeat it a few times to get it into your account. Having the changes in your life can take a few times and a few days or weeks, but they will come if you do this treatment, as mentioned. Now I can hear you say, "if I can do all of this myself, why would I go to a hypnotherapist?"

Here is a reply.

The terms hypnosis and hypnotherapist distinguish significantly. One is a mind-state, and one is therapy.

Self-hypnosis can do a lot of good. There are many things you can learn with self-hypnosis. There's one extremely important thing that you can't do with self-hypnosis, which is treatment.

A hypnotherapist uses therapeutic tools to make changes in their lives while the client is in a state of Hypnosis. It is not possible for someone in Hypnosis to ask questions and dig far more in-depth and use the tools necessary to discover the root of a problem or engage in a healing method with their inner child.

Self-hypnosis is of exceptional value for minimizing stress and other associated issues. Having a hypnotherapist to deal with to get to the root of a problem and find solutions is vital to a healing experience.

When you try to find a hypnotherapist, discover someone you feel comfortable with. Ensure that they do the work with the training. Test their credentials where possible. Any governmental organization does not govern hypnotherapy, and anybody can hang a shingle and call themselves a hypnotherapist. Make sure that the person you are working with is well educated and professional in their field of operation. This is much easier to take your time in finding the best hypnotherapist in advance than you later discover that you have messed up.

HYPNOSIS TRUTH

Others can only imagine the zombie-like hypnotic trances in the Hollywood movies we see! Others may have appeared to be using Hypnosis to the typical areas such as dropping weight and giving up cigarette smoking.

Yet it can shock a lot of you to read this that the American Medical Association has approved Hypnosis for use in healthcare facilities given that as long ago as the late 1950s! And every week, it seems like there are brand-new findings and outcomes from brand-new studies showing the hypnosis effectiveness.

I know you will find that incredibly open-minded and very interesting! So, let's go in, are we going to?

• 'Hypnotherapists possess special powers!'

Don't let it be! Of course, they can produce some strong results, but it's not as cape and dagger or magical as all those old Hollywood movies will have us believe!

The therapists have no special abilities at all. They just have the expertise and experience to help get you into a heightened state of relaxation, and then provide your inner mind with the best kind of message, which puts thought into action!

• "Hypnosis deals only with the poor minded people!"

It is the ones who can concentrate and have a more imaginative mind with Hypnosis that gets the best results.

That's because all the Hypnosis is Hypnosis in itself. And with that technique and skillset, those individuals with higher concentration and creativity have even more efficient outcomes.

Hypnosis has also been used by thousands around the world to enhance trust and self-confidence, release dependencies, release when crippling fears and phobias, eventually lose that weight, stop smoking cigarettes, increase mental capacity, and the list continues.

Chapter 2: HOW HYPNOSIS WORKS AND WHAT IT IMPLIES

In 1891, the British Medical Association voted for the use of Hypnosis in medication; but, until 1955, years later, it was not approved! It has helped to address various issues such as; weight management, cigarette smoking addiction, exercise motivation, improving research study patterns, controlling stressing behaviors, and maintaining good self-esteem are, however, a few of the conditions that can be affected by healing Hypnosis, with positive results.

Let me now put some of your potential worries to rest and erase from your mind any of the doubts you might have.

Hypnosis will only occur if you like it. You can only be hypnotized if you enable it. I can't address you directly and captivate you without encouraging you to understand. This means that Hypnosis is healthy for someone who wants to help with it and more!

Hypnosis is not some sort of magical control of the mind that robs you of your will or ability to make educated decisions.

Hypnosis is a transformed state of consciousness that makes you more receptive to suggestions and directions that are intended to help you make favorable mental and physical improvement crazies such as weight management, cigarette smoking addiction, exercise encouragement, boost research habits, manage worried activities and develop healthy self-confidence. With a wide spectrum of mental and physical disorders, it is only one of the many treatment strategies that can help in a long-range way.

You can't be forced to do anything against your will or your ethical code under Hypnosis. It occurs during the session, which requires your immediate attention; you will still be able to deal with it.

You may not accept that you stay in a hypnotic trance during your hypnosis session, but you should be able to note your concentration tightly, and you are breathing steadily as you begin to reach the alpha and relax.

Alpha is a level of consciousness or a hypnotic coma, referred to as the Beta state of consciousness, which is one level mentioned below as being wide-awake or fully aware. You may become a hundred times more sensitive to suggestions and guidance in the Alpha state as an essentially conscious individual, or the Beta state.

There is a pathway passing straight through the conscious through the subconscious mind to explain the advantages of the Alpha state, imagine. Such suggestions are 200 times more likely to be accurate in the subconscious than the things we say to ourselves in our usual Beta state. Hypnosis is a method of rearranging connections in mind in more desirable and safer directions.

In some situations, with weight management, we need to look a little further into finding the root cause of the weight gain, and this could take additional sessions; however, the outcomes at the end will warrant spending this extra time. An American Health Magazine report showed that after 600 sessions, psychoanalysis provided a 38 percent recovery, behavioral therapy provided a 72 percent recovery after 22 sessions. After six sessions, hypnosis provided a phenomenal 93 percent cure. As you can see, Hypnosis has proven to be very effective and safe in helping you reach your goals quickly.

Hypnose is a safe condition. It is something you experience daily. For example, you 're in a state of Hypnosis when you're absorbed by an excellent picture of motion or a TV show. You've experienced Hypnosis if you've ever been driving to work or the shop and questioned how you got there because your mind was considering a thousand other things. You have been in a trance if you've ever been in the "forest" where you're focused on the job at hand and nothing else. If you've ever found yourself dreaming for the day, you've been in hypnosis.

You can also be so distracted when you are reading a good book that you don't hear when anyone is talking to you. Then, the brain is in a different state-hypnosis. However, doing things like watching movies or reading outstanding books isn't needed. This can even be irritating stuff that places you in a hypnotic state, like an awkward lecture. If someone is speaking in a monotonous voice, remaining focused can be difficult. You could start dreaming about something more exciting that's Hypnosis as well.

Have in mind that you might be conscious of everything I say during the session, and that's cool because you're still in Hypnosis, you can constantly get back to the waking Beta state by opening your eyes or counting "ONE-TWO-THREE" in your head, and above all, you 're still in charge.

Why consider Hypnosis?

Hypnosis is commonly used to deal with several conditions in situations with unsafe drugs. But what is used to treat anesthesia? Hypnosis can be used as a single or in combination with other therapies.

Chapter 3: IMPROVE YOUR EATING HABITS WITH HYPNOSIS

The first move to use weight loss hypnosis: Recognizing why you are not meeting your goals. How's this working out? A hypnotherapist will typically ask you questions about your weight loss, i.e., about your eating habits and exercise habits.

This gathering of information helps to identify what you might need to help with the work.

You will then be directed through induction, a method of calming the mind and body, and entering a hypnosis state. Your mind is highly suggestible while in hypnosis. You've lost your aware and rational mind – so the hypnotherapist will talk to your unconscious thoughts directly.

The hypnotherapist will give you positive suggestions, affirmations in hypnosis and may ask you to visualize the changes. With our many recordings of weight loss hypnosis, you can try this right now! Positive weight-loss hypnosis suggestions could include:

Making morale higher: Positive comments will improve your sense of trust by promoting words.

Visualization of Success: You may be asked during hypnosis to visualize meeting your weight loss goals and the way it makes you feel.

Reframing the Identity inside: Hypnosis will help you control an inner voice that "doesn't want" to give up unhealthy food and turn it into an ally on your weight loss journey that is fast and more logical with constructive suggestions.

Tapping the Aware: In the hypnotic state, the unconscious patterns which lead to unhealthy eating can begin to be identified. In other words, you will become more conscious of why we make poor food decisions and portion control and develop more conscientious food decision strategies.

Fending Anxiety Off Hypnotic advice will help calm the fear of struggling to achieve weight loss. Fear is the number one reason people may never get going in the first place.

The detection and reframing of habits pattern: When you are in hypnosis, you can analyze and discover how you use such unconscious reactions to eat, and "turn off." We can start slowing down by repeated positive affirmations and ultimately completely remove automatic, unconscious thought.

Developing new strategies for coping: Hypnosis helps you to develop better ways to deal with tension, emotions, and relationships. You might be asked to view a stressful situation, for example, and then visualize yourself with a healthy snack to respond.

Rehearsing Eating Good: You may be asked to rehearse making healthy eating choices during hypnosis, i.e., being OK with taking food home at a restaurant. It tends to make healthier decisions more automatic. Rehearsal helps in managing cravings, too.

Make dietary options healthier: You will love unhealthy foods and want them. Hypnosis can help you begin to develop a taste or desire for healthy choices, and can also affect the portion sizes you select.

Rising Indications Unconscious: You may have learned, through repetition, to drown out the signals that your body sends when you feel full. Hypnotherapy allows you to become more conscious of those metrics.

Naturally, not every suggestion applies to you. The hypnotherapy program-whether you work with a hypnotherapist or self-hypnosis-should include ideas specific to the food relationship. For example, Clara (from the above example) may focus on teaching the unconscious to slow down their automatic responses, as well as providing the unconscious with new, more effective ways of handling stress.

Working with a certified hypnotherapist may help you to refine your strategy to suit your specific needs.

How hypnotherapy can help you to lose weight

In the hypnotic state, your mind is considerably more open to suggestion. Research has shown that during hypnosis, several fascinating changes occur in your brain, which helps you to learn without objectively thinking about the knowledge you are getting.

Which is to say, you are disconnected from the rational mind. Therefore the vital conscious mind does not doubt what you think when you receive hypnotic suggestions.

Repetition, however, is key to performance. That is why, after an initial visit, most hypnotherapists send you home with self-hypnosis recordings. In your mind, the barriers are high. Only through repeated work can you untangle those convictions successfully and reframe them.

But hearing repeated statements and encouraging ideas about healthy eating is a first step in the process of weight loss. You 're teaching people to think differently. Yet those assertions will support you:

Control Craving

Even if you can remove yourself from the cravings? Isolate them, and dispatch them? Hypnosis techniques for certain weight loss help you do this. For example, you might be asked to visualize sending your cravings away – say out to sea on a ship. Suggestions will also help you to reframe your cravings, and learn how to control them better.

Expect Success

Reality dictates expectations. Naturally, when we expect success, we are more likely to take the required steps to achieve that success. Hypnotherapy for weight loss will plant the seed of success in your subconscious, which can be a strong unconscious motivator to keep you on track.

Practice Positivity

Negativity too much spoils weight loss. There are foods that you can't consume. Unhealthy food "kills" you. Hypnotherapy allows one to reframe these ideas in a more optimistic way-you don't starve yourself; you shed what you don't need.

Ready for Relapse

We've been conditioned to believe there are humiliating relapses – excuses to give up. Yet hypnosis tells us to think differently about a relapse. A relapse is an opportunity to analyze what went wrong, learn from it, and be better prepared to be tempted.

Transform your behavior

One small step at a time achieves big goals. Hypnotherapy empowers us to make small changes that feed into larger objectives. Say you 're rewarding yourself with sugary, high-calorie foods; you might be working on choosing a healthier reward through hypnosis.

Visualize Success

Hypnotic vision, at last, is a strong motivator. Visualization helps you to "see" consequences and discuss how they make you feel. You could also visualize your future-self, saying you have what it takes to succeed.

Research Review: Weight loss hypnosis

Will it work with hypnosis? That is a question that anyone who considers hypnotherapy has – and it's a question that has been interested in research for decades.

The work appears to paint an optimistic picture of the efficacy of hypnotherapy. Several studies have shown that hypnosis can lead to weight loss in the long term and that hypnosis experiences higher success levels compared to conventional weight loss methods.

A 1985 study-one of the first to look at hypnosis of weight loss-compared two classes. One party changed the diet and started exercising; the other did the same, but also provided hypnotherapy. The hypnosis group had retained or improved weight loss after eight months, and two years-the the other groups had lost much of the back weight.

Similarly, a report in 1986 looked at 60 women overweight by 20 percent. The hypnosis group lost 17 pounds after six months, while the non-hypnosis community lost just half a pound.

A 1996 meta-analysis looked at the effect of adding hypnosis to treatments for weight loss. What the researchers found was compelling: Hypnosis nearly doubled the weight loss during treatment. And hypnosis increased efficacy by 146 percent after treatment.

More recently, a study in 2014 showed that hypnosis has several positive weight-loss effects. Participants undergoing hypnosis reduced weight and BMI, as well as changed dietary habits. Another gain found in the analysis was enhanced body image.

Starting with Weight Loss Hypnosis

Are you ready to begin your journey into weight loss? You've got many different options to get started. For face-to-face sessions, you can visit a licensed hypnotherapist. Having a hypnotherapist, you can schedule a virtual conference. Other options include recorded hypnosis or self-hypnosis. All of the methods showed promise for weight loss.

One-on-one hypnosis — A hypnotherapist will help you to identify the unconscious barriers which hold you back. Plus, a hypnotherapist will help you to overcome certain issues in hypnosis sessions. These can be carried out at the office or via video conferencing.

Guided hypnosis — A guided recording of hypnosis can help you get started quickly and learn the techniques of hypnosis at home or on the go. These are recordings of licensed hypnotherapists who guide you through induction and then offer constructive feedback through the recording.

Self-Hypnosis — Individuals play the position of hypnotherapists in self-hypnosis, use a memorized script to trigger hypnosis, and offer constructive advice.

Who should try Weight Loss Hypnosis?

The perfect candidate is, frankly, someone who has difficulty sticking to a balanced diet and workout routine because their bad patterns don't seem to shake, Gurniak says. It's a sign of a subconscious problem to get trapped in unhealthy habits — like eating the entire bag of potato chips instead of stopping when you're finished.

Your subconscious, Friedmutter notes, is where your thoughts, behaviors, and addictions reside. And since hypnotherapy is treating the subconscious, rather than just the conscious, it can be more successful. Indeed, a 1970 research review showed that hypnosis had a success rate of 93 percent, with fewer sessions required than both psychotherapy and behavioral therapy. "This prompted researchers to conclude that hypnosis was the most powerful tool for modifying attitudes, thought patterns, and behavior," Friedmutter says.

Neither can hypnotherapy be used on its own. Gurniak says hypnosis can also be used as a complement to other weight loss programs designed by professionals to treat different conditions of health, be it diabetes, obesity, arthritis, or cardiovascular disease.

What should I expect while I am being treated?

Depending on the practitioner, the sessions can vary in length and methodology. For example, Dr. Cruz says that her sessions typically last between 45 and 60 minutes, while Friedmutter sees patients with a weight loss for three to four hours. But generally speaking, you can expect to lie down, relax with your eyes closed, and let the hypnotherapist guide you through specific techniques and suggestions that can help you achieve your goals.

"The aim is to train the mind to move toward the good and away from the unhealthy," says Friedmutter. "I'm able to determine subconscious hitches through client history that sent the client off their original [health] blueprint. Just as we learn to use food to abuse our bodies, we can learn to honor them.'

Nd no, you 're not going to cluck like a chicken or confess deep, dark secrets. "You can't get stuck in hypnosis, or have something said or done against your will," says Gurniak. "If it's contrary to your values or convictions, you 're not going to act on the information provided during the trance."

Instead, you'll probably experience deep relaxation while still being aware of what's being said, adds Gurniak. "It would describe someone in a hypnotic trance as being wide awake and asleep in between," he says. "They are fully in control at all times and able to stop the process, because you can only be hypnotized if you choose to. We function as a team to achieve the goal of the person.

Naturally, the number of sessions you need depends entirely on your response to the hypnosis. Some might see outcomes as little as one to three, says Dr. Cruz, while others would require from eight to fifteen sessions elsewhere. And then again, this may not be effective for all.

Chapter 4: SELF-HYPNOSIS TO RELEASE BAD EATING HABITS

When it comes to hypnotherapy, people have some options: one-on-one sessions with a hypnotherapist, listening to recordings of hypnosis, and self-hypnosis. Self-hypnosis is one of the most convenient, because you can use it at home or the office.

Food addictions are also highly recommended. To learn how to use Grace's self-hypnosis, check out this video. As you can see, that is a simple operation. Here are a few things you may want to bear in mind:

Note Your Well-being: How is it that you feel? Assessing how you feel is helpful so at the end of the session you can reassess it.

Controlled Breathing and Visualization: Deep breathing shows that relaxation is time for the body and mind. Visualization is also another form of relaxation initiation.

A Guided Countdown: You can countdown from 10 to pick. This helps the mind enter a hypnosis-state.

Strong affirmations: You should talk directly to the subconscious when you're comfortable. Offer affirmations to it, constructive ideas for reconditioning the mind. With food addiction, for instance, you might repeat something like: "I 'm free from overeating. I listen to know my body when to eat. I prefer to eat full portions of nutritious foods. I'm avoiding sugary foods. Every single day, I feel healthier.

Visualizing the Change: Visualize the way you will be following the healthier path after you have given your subconscious positive suggestions. See yourself living on a balanced food partnership. This strengthens the idea and allows it to take hold and to sustain it.

Hypnotherapy and aversion therapy: reframing the mind

Sweet, salty, or fatty foods bring with them several side effects.

Overindulgence is linked to obesity, diabetes, energy shortages, and even depression. This leads to productivity losses, a lower sex drive and, to name a few, anxiety. But still, we are obligated to consume these foods.

What if we could help the mind avoid craving for unhealthy foods? What if we didn't tell the mind when we saw a brownie or chocolate cake that I want to eat a lot of that?

Well, aversion hypnosis is one strategy which is offered by trained hypnotherapists that can help us do just that. It's not always necessary but it's often one of the most effective solutions for food addiction.

To tell the truth, we aren't big fans of aversion therapy for most topics (we'd rather focus our customers on what they want, like a slim healthy body, rather than a negative version of what they don't want, like a cake covered in ants), but when it comes to food and sugar, we find that aversion therapy can be so helpful in tipping the scales for customers that we have to include it here as a possible solution.

Aversion therapy, while creating positive associations with the better option, allows us to create negative associations with something. A hypnotherapist may begin by saying the food is life. Food is natural and derived from nature.

Instead, they might establish a derogatory junk food association (i.e., it's detrimental to us, or even it's poison to our bodies).

Remember: The subconscious desires that we feel safe. So when we eat sugary, fatty snacks and light up those reward centers, the subconscious feels we've been given a favor. But it didn't.

Why not for the subconscious, simply? Take the mind away from thinking of processed foods as a reward, or as a comfort blanket – but as a dangerous and unhealthy choice.

Does Food Addictions Hypnosis Work? What Does Research Say

Much of the work on food addiction hypnosis or hypnosis for stopping sugar was conducted around weight loss. And the report is crystal clear. Hypnosis has proved a powerful tool to help people lose weight.

Yes, one study showed that those who used hypnosis on average suffered 20 percent more than those who did not. Additional studies have also found hypnosis to contribute to longer-term outcomes for healthy eating.

Hypnosis has a significant weight loss impact

Researchers investigated how hypnosis could help 60 attendees lose weight in 1986. Hypnosis was used to support ego-strengthening, decision-making, and motivation in the participants. The group that used hypnosis, or 17 pounds to just 0.5 pounds, lost 30 times more on average. (To know more, review our weight loss hypnosis blog!)

Hypnosis The loss of more than 90 percent of others

A meta-analysis of weight loss hypnosis research analyzed 18 studies contrasting cognitive behavioral therapy – i.e. relaxation preparation and controlled imaging – with the same hypnosis-complemented therapies. The results: Hypnosis has helped people lose weight and keep off the weight. Many subjects with hypnosis lost more than 90% of the non-hypnosis community and held it off for two years.

Hypnosis Long Term Weight Loss

One research looked at how hypnosis improved a weight-management treatment plan. 109 participants completed a therapeutic plan in the study, with or without hypnosis. Both groups had lost significant weight after 9 weeks. Yet the hypnosis group tended to lose considerable weight at the 8-month and 2-year follow-ups, and it managed to achieve its weight targets.

Start your journey to hypnosis today

Much of the work on food addiction hypnosis or hypnosis for stopping sugar was conducted around weight loss. And the report is crystal clear. Hypnosis has proved a powerful tool to help people lose weight.

Yes, one study showed that those who used hypnosis on average suffered 20 percent more than those who did not. Additional studies have also found hypnosis to contribute to longer-term outcomes for healthy eating.

Hypnosis has a significant weight loss impact

Researchers investigated how hypnosis could help 60 attendees lose weight in 1986. Hypnosis was used to support ego-strengthening, decision-making, and motivation in the participants. The group that used hypnosis, or 17 pounds to just 0.5 pounds, lost 30 times more on average. (To know more, review our weight loss hypnosis blog!)

Hypnosis The loss of more than 90 percent of others

A meta-analysis of weight loss hypnosis research analyzed 18 studies contrasting cognitive behavioral therapy – i.e. relaxation preparation and controlled imaging – with the same hypnosis-complemented therapies. The results: Hypnosis has helped people lose weight and keep off the weight. Many subjects with hypnosis lost more than 90% of the non-hypnosis community and held it off for two years.

Hypnosis Long Term Weight Loss

If you could avoid emotional eating now, what would make your life differently?

Would anyone else notice, or are they just you?

You may wonder how this situation got you. In your mind, you know full well that food is the only thing to do when you 're hungry.

Every other creature on this earth and you know this. It's our way of surviving. You know that eating food when you're not hungry is a formula for discomfort, shame, diminished self-esteem, and weight gain, of course, not just in your brain.

Stop emotional eating? How did it kick-off?

How is it that humans, alone among all the thousands of species of creatures that exist, often seek to fulfill needs that have little to do with bodily hunger for food?

To feel irritated, so instead of coping with what upsets them, head for some pizza in the kitchen. Feeling lonely and mumming on a candy bar instead of finding more social ties. What's the point?

Okay, it is partially because we are so smart. (Ironic, do you not believe?)

We are also the only creatures that use symbols (as far as we know). One thing we can do is stand for another. This is a brilliant skill, and it has allowed us to develop highly sophisticated societies, and to do things that should be very difficult for us on the face of it. But we can and do use the symbols in both negative and positive ways.

This is what happens when we feel an emotional pang, which is like a hunger pang in some ways, so we get somehow reminded of the comfort that comes from eating when we're hungry. Then we make that 'eating comfort' stand-in for whatever it is that would satisfy that emotional need, without really thinking too hard about it. And we're eating.

Tackling the question correctly

You 're going to hear about those horrible feelings of remorse that afflict you after you've indulged in such emotional eating, as though you've done something wrong and you're a bad person somehow. But the culpability is also a consequence of misuse of symbols. It stands in for the real problem, which is that it is not meeting some important needs of yours.

You say this is all very well and very interesting, but how do I get out of it? I did not consciously plan to start eating like this, but I don't seem to be able to stop it, even though I want to!

Hypnosis can help you change old habits

Stop Emotional Eating is a powerful session of audio hypnosis that can help you lose weight and maintain a healthier lifestyle by breaking the grip of this pattern of behavior at the level where it was established-in your unconscious mind.

As you relax and listen to your download over and over again, you will notice several subtle yet significant changes taking place. This you'll find:

Your mind is clearer and your feelings calmer every time you relax and allow yourself this private time.

You are learning a powerful way of changing the way negative experiences influence you in the present

It begins to feel quite normal to keep the emotional needs and physical needs in your mind very apart-from what you are doing. You begin to find creative ways to deal more effectively with your emotional needs. Eating healthier every day feels natural and normal. You start feeling very good about yourself

hypnotherapy Weight loss

Our specialty is hypnosis for weight loss. When the permanent weight loss procedure of the Gastric Mind Band was introduced over ten years ago, this was to provide a clear alternative to the gastric surgical band.

People who are overweight are increasingly searching for solutions to help them on their weight loss journey, but many are reluctant to go for typical gastric band procedures to help build a better relationship with food. Consequently, gastric band hypnosis provides a feasible option, which is healthy and very inexpensive.

Hypnotherapy for weight loss along with gastric band hypnosis has become increasingly common and widely available in recent years. People know the many distinct, beneficial effects of hypnotherapy and are therefore much less cynical about these forms of treatments. Let us make it clear at the outset, however, that the Gastric Mind Band Permanent Weight Loss treatment plan, as provided at the Elite Clinic, does not rely solely on hypnosis; it is certainly not what you would normally define as hypnosis of the gastric bands.

Weight loss hypnosis: Explained

Hypnosis is a state of mind that happens naturally; it is the same state of deep relaxation that you feel when you are about to fall asleep at night. It may also happen while you're dreaming, listening to music or watching a very good movie: when you're concentrating deeply on something important, you can be unaware of what's going on around you, or how much time has gone by.

Gastric band hypnotherapy is the therapeutic use of hypnosis, which is typically carried out in a psychiatric setting to help people make meaningful changes that progress in different areas of their lives. Worded ideas are used by a hypnotherapist to help you solve particular challenges, such as modifying and breaking an unhelpful habit, such as smoking or even chewing your nails. Hypnotherapy can also be used to help you relinquish negative thoughts, build a more optimistic self-image, increase self-esteem, and improve self-assurance.

And how does hypnotherapy, this weight loss, work in the weight loss field? Research results often support the claim that using hypnotherapy/hypnosis in the area of weight loss can be highly effective and help to build a better relationship with your food, in fact in terms of success it is comparable with the gastric band. You can read the abstracts Hypnosis efficacy as an adjunct to behavioral weight management, as well as hypnotherapy controlled trial for weight loss in patients with obstructive sleep apnoea.

Overeating hypnosis: Get over your sugar addiction

Do you find yourself reaching during the day for snacks, or at mealtime for extra portions? We 're all doing the same. There comes a point, though, when the habit becomes unhealthy.

Do you want to make a change and end your overeating?

Participants who had hypnosis for overeating reported significant additional weight loss relative to the control group during this study.

Get set to hear more about hypnotic binge feeding! This guide discusses everything you need to decide if hypnotherapy is right for you. Start jumping in and stop your binge eating habit today!

How to confess your food addiction

For overheating, let's think about food addiction before you get a taste of the information around hypnosis. Disordered eating is when you have formed an unhealthy diet- and eating relationship.

Here are some symptoms to watch for that will help you decide whether you have an addiction to food.

Pressure & Never ending worry

We've all felt pressure — by both the media and our peers — to look at a certain way. Sticking to unrealistic beauty standards, however, can have an impact on your health. You can feel forced to diet, which may lead to anxiety and binge eating.

You may also feel constantly concerned about dieting, eating, and exercising.

If you feel ashamed or guilty about how much you eat, this can add unnecessary pressure to your life.

From dieting to eating disorders

When people feel pressured to look some way by the media, they begin dieting.

But dieting will leave you worrying about food. You can develop disordered eating habits or an eating disorder as a result. This will commit you to a constant diet/binge eating cycle.

The Lasting Process

You'll probably establish an unhealthy eating habit when you become obsessed with food and weight loss. This pattern will leave you constraining yourself, missing meals, eating binge, and then dieting again.

You'll notice constant fluctuations in your weight as you diet yo-yo.

In time, in this endless loop, you might feel like yourself trapped.

The Symptoms

While several different eating disorders occur, the general symptoms include:

- Eating food too quickly
- Continue eating, even if you're full
- Hiding food or feeding in silence
- Feeling forced to eat
- Felt bad after consuming too much

- Eat when you don't feel hungry

Hold your mind on those signs. Hypnotherapy for overeating habits may help if you believe you have a food addiction.

Overeating Hypnosis: How It Works

So, does hypnosis work for overeating?

Yeah! According to this report, patients undergoing overeating hypnotherapy demonstrated greater progress than at least 70 percent of nonhypnotic care clients.

Hypnotherapy will help you conquer an addiction to food. Here are a few ways in which hypnotherapy can help stop us from eating too much.

Mindful Eating

Food addictions cause people to over-eat with little thought. When we fail to think about our actions it becomes a compulsion.

Hypnosis can teach the mind to stay conscious.

You'll learn how to know your cravings, how full you are already feeling, and how to keep your eating conscious. Mindfulness should make you aware of your actions so that when you feed, you will gain control over how often you consume and how much you feed.

Habit breakers

We develop habitual thinking over time. Binge eating causes us to talk to negative, harmful thoughts about ourselves. We end up eating binge again in response, triggering a relentless cycle of binge eating.

These negative thoughts can cause our cravings, overeating and stress.

Take a breath during those moments and remember that everything is okay. Otherwise, the stress becomes anxiety and encourages your binge eating.

To end your food addiction you must break these negative spirals of thought.

Overeating hypnosis will help you break the habit.

You will take charge of your emotions by using hypnosis. Rather than swimming in the negatives, you'll learn how to make your subconscious a friend (not an enemy).

Treat the Base Condition

Food dependency is often triggered by another disorder.

You could have depression or an anxiety disorder, for example. Such conditions may cause you to think negatively, which in turn encourages your binge eating.

Hypnosis can empower you and give you the strength of mind you need to fight these conditions. You should take charge and adjust the script, instead of allowing your depression or anxiety to dominate your thoughts.

Treating the underlying disorder will help you break your eating binge habits.

Restore Your Faith

A lack of confidence in oneself can cause us to freeze. Instead of acting or managing our negative feelings, we believe like something is beyond our control.

When we lack self-confidence our negative thoughts can take over.

Hypnotherapy will help you develop faith in yourself. You can take back control by learning how to believe in yourself. Thus, you can end your unhealthy eating binge habits.

With overeating hypnotherapy, you will have the confidence to surmount anything.

Techniques for Self-Hypnosis

You should know that you have a few choices available before you continue using hypnotherapy for overeating. For example, one-on-one sessions with a hypnotherapist may be considered. You can also want to listen to the tapes for hypnotherapy.

There is self-hypnosis, as well. Here are some techniques to help get you started:

- ✓ Note your wellbeing and assess how you feel at the start and end of each session
- ✓ Breathe in to tell your mind and body that it is time to relax
- ✓ Count down from 10 which tells your mind that you are in a hypnosis state
- ✓ Talk to yourself using affirmations or constructive advice like "I'm free to over-eat"
- ✓ Imagine taking control of yourself and living a happier, healthier life
- ✓ You can relax with these techniques, and reframe your mind. Application of overeating hypnosis will help you regain control of your eating patterns and daily life.'
- ✓ Binge Eating and Food Addiction hypnotherapy: How it can help

But just how does that work?

Here's a look at some of the finer binge eating and food addiction hypnosis points, and some of the many ways it can empower us to lead healthier lives.

Mindful Eating:

Nearly all food addictions have a common symptom: Overeating sometimes without thought. It is becoming a habit, and something we don't even think about.

They will train the mind to be more conscious of our cravings, how full they feel, and the actual act of eating with hypnosis for mindful feeding. Mindful eating hypnosis allows us to recognize hunger cravings and physical feelings, and to be thoughtful about eating. We are gaining control over food and our cravings.

Breaking Popular Thoughts:

All too often habitual thinking becomes reactionary and negative. And those thoughts also cause overeating or craving.

You may encounter a stressful situation at work and instead of taking a breath and saying it's all going to be Fine, you start feeling you 're underqualified or the stress turns to anxiety.

We can't overcome our food addictions without stopping the spiraling thought patterns.

Hypnosis empowers you to take control of our minds and make a strong friend of our subconscious.

Underlying Conditions to Repair:

Any number of factors can trigger binge eating: Depression, anxiety, lack of self-love, to name a few. Hypnosis can empower us to manage those conditions and move past them.

Restoring Faith:

Lack of self-confidence or love can stop us from acting. If we don't trust ourselves, or if we don't value ourselves, then we can allow our bad habits to continue.

Hypnotherapy is a strong instrument for gaining confidence and learning to love ourselves more. This is important about food addictions. We are much more likely to experience cravings when we love and believe in ourselves and work towards making healthy lifestyle choices.

Chapter 5: GASTRIC BAND HYPNOTHERAPY AS AN APPROACH TO WEIGHT LOSS

Losing weight when you're tempted or no will power isn't an easy way to go. Still, if you're trying to lose weight just to add up more pounds, then you can think about losing weight the healthy way, use the Virtual Gastric Band method with the well-known health expert Claire Hegarty as seen on television and often heard on the radio.

Claire Hegarty, a leader in the field of Virtual Gastric Band Hypnotherapy and Gastric Band Hypnosis, not only offers you Gastric Band Hypnotherapy but also offers you a new technique called TranceBand (R) which is Gastric Band Hypnotherapy, Timeline Therapy, Food Education as well as other techniques and services to deliver powerful weight loss outcomes.

Using Hypnosis, NLP, EFT, and CBT strategies, a virtual gastric band lets you slim out. The techniques of Hypnosis Weight Loss allow you to be reassured that you are fitted with a gastric band where you will have all the sensations without the risk and pain an Invasive Gastric Band Operation will bring, and you will still lose weight.

The virtual gastric band offers real results

Claire Hegarty Hypnotherapy Gastric Band gives you real performance. Here are some of the benefits which a Hypnotherapy Virtual Gastric Band can bring:

1. There is no invasive Surgery with a Virtual Gastric Band
2. No fear of getting an operation to have a gastric band fitted
3. No Comfort With Virtual Gastric Band
4. Virtual gastric bands are considerably more cost-effective
5. No Time off work fitted with a virtual gastric band
6. No Complications of gastric bands with surgery

THE DIFFERENCE BETWEEN STAGE SHOWS AND HYPNOSIS

Certain people get confused when it comes to the treatment of the Hypnotic Gastric Band. When we talk about the Hypnotic Gastric Band and hypnotherapy some people immediately think about stage hypnosis where famous stage hypnosis performers get people to do dumb things for the entertainment of others, the technique of the Hypnotic Gastric Band isn't like that.

Looking at this stage hypnosis shows you think it's the stage hypnotherapist who makes these people do stupid things, you think people do things they don't want to do, and the hypnotherapist is controlling them, but that's not the case.

The stage hypnotist calls for volunteers to go up on stage, you'll find that the volunteers are exhibitionists who immediately stand up to ask to be a part of the act. These volunteers are the kind of people you can recall at school who loved being the center of attention and who was always playing around in the classroom, these volunteers like to stand out from the crowd and love to behave differently or stupidly in those situations.

The stage hypnotist will do a variety of tests to make sure he has selected the right kind of people; he will want to ensure that he has people who are most suggestible and who will do well for the crowd.

And as you can see, the hypnotic gastric band technique is completely different; you are not there to perform, you are using a hypnotic gastric band specialist to support you to lose weight, no one can make you do something that you do not want to do.

Stage hypnosis is entirely different from regular hypnotherapy, such as the weight reduction treatment with the hypnotic gastric band.

Does Gastric Band Hypnosis involve surgery?

This is a popular question people wonder about the technique of the Hypno Gastric Band, and the answer is No! The Hypno Gastric Band requires no surgery and instead uses methods of hypnotherapy, which also includes cognitive behavioral therapy and nutritional education.

Is the treatment for the gastric band hypnosis a painful one?

The gastric band Hypnosis is in no way unpleasant. Instead, you're left to feel relaxed and comfortable in the full knowledge that you have a professional Hypnosis Gastric Band working with you to help you lose weight in a healthy and controlled way.

I have Heard That Gastric Bypass Procedure Can Have Complications, Are There Complications Involved in The Gastric Band Technique Hypnotherapy?

There are no complications involved with Gastric Band Hypnotherapy, leaving you aware that using Claire Hegarty's Hypnosis Gastric Band procedure is a safe way to become the real you and lose the weight you want to lose.

Will I be aware of what is happening when I am hypnotized?

People get confused with Stage Hypnosis and having hypnosis with a weight-loss professional. When you see Claire Hegarty as part of your technique for the Hypnosis Gastric Band, when you're hypnotized, you'll feel calm and relaxed and be in complete control, knowing exactly what's going on.

EVERYTHING YOU NEED TO KNOW ABOUT WEIGHT LOSS HYPNOSIS AND GASTRIC BAND

Hypnosis might be best known as the party trick used to make people do the chicken dance on stage, but more and more people turn to mind-control techniques to help them make healthier choices and lose weight. Case in point: The dieting veteran turned to Hypnosis when Georgia, 28, realized she had to lose the 30 or so pounds she put on following foot surgery in 2009. In the past, the mind-control method had helped her resolve a fear of flight, and she hoped that this would also help her create healthier eating habits.

At first, the self-proclaimed foodie was taken aback by the recommendations of her hypnotherapist. "[She had] four basic agreements that I will have to stick to: eat when you're hungry, listen to your body and eat whatever you want, stop when you're full, eat slowly and enjoy every bite," explains Georgia. "As such, no meal was off-limits, and I was allowed to eat all to my ears in moderation-music!"

Who To Try Hypnosis

Hypnosis is a way of losing weight and making healthy eating a habit for anyone looking for a gentle way to. Isn't it for one person? Anyone wants a fast fix. It takes time to reframe problematic thoughts about food-Georgia tells her hypnotherapist eight times a year, and it took a month before she started to notice a real change. "The weight slowly and steadily fell without any drastic changes in my lifestyle. I was still dining out several times a week, but also sent meals back with food on them!

It's very good not to think of hypnosis as a diet at all, says Joshua E. Syna, MA, LCDC, a Houston Hypnosis Center accredited hypnotherapist. "It works because it alters their way of thinking about nutrition and food, and it helps them to learn to be calmer and more comfortable in their lives. So instead of nutrition and eating as an emotional response, it becomes a suitable solution to hunger, and new patterns of behavior are being formed that help the person to cope with emotions and life," he explains. "Hypnosis works for weight loss as it allows the individual to separate food and eat from their emotional life."

Dr. Stein says the use of at-home self-guided audio programs created by a professional hypnotist (look for an ASCH certification) is good for people with no other mental health problems. But beware of all the latest online consumer applications-one study found that most applications are untested and sometimes make grandiose statements about their efficacy, which can not be substantiated.

What Does Hypnosis Feel Like

Forget what you've seen in films, and on stage, therapeutic hypnosis is closer than a circus trick to a therapy session. "Hypnosis is a collaborative process and every step of the way the patient should be well educated and relaxed," says Dr. Stein. And she adds to people concerned about being fooled into doing something strange or dangerous, even under hypnosis if you don't want to do it, you won't. "It's concentrated attention, really," she says.

"Naturally, everyone goes into light trance statements several times a day-think of when you zone out when a friend shares every aspect of their holidays-and hypnosis is only learning to concentrate your internal attention beneficially."

Dispelling the myth from the patient's side that hypnosis feels weird or scary, Georgia says she's always felt very lucid and under control. There were also funny moments like when the vision of walking on the scale and seeing the target weight was told. "My overly creative mind had to imagine first removing all the clothes, every bit of jewelry, my watch, and hair clip before jumping on in the nude. Anyone else does that, or is it just me?"

THE ONE DOWNSIDE TO WEIGHT LOSS HYPNOSIS

This isn't harmful; this combines well with other therapies for weight loss and needs no tablets, powders, or other supplements. Nothing happens at the very worst, putting it in the camp of 'might help, can't hurt.' But Dr. Stein admits there is one downside: quality. Costs per hour vary depending on your location, but for therapeutic hypnosis treatments, it ranges from $100 to $250 an hour, and when you see the therapist for a month or two, once a week or more, that can add up quickly.

And most insurance companies do not support the hypnosis. However, Dr. Stein says it can be covered if used as part of a bigger mental health therapy plan, so check with your provider.

A Stunning Weight Loss Hypnosis Perk

Hypnosis is not just a mental thing, there's also a medical component, says Peter LePort, MD, a bariatric surgeon and MemorialCare Center for Obesity medical director in California. "You have to deal with any underlying weight gain metabolic or biological causes first, but while you're doing that using hypnosis can kick-off healthy habits," he says. And there is another healthy benefit of using hypnosis: "The aspect of meditation can help to reduce stress and increase awareness, which can also help with weight loss," he adds.

So Hypnosis Works Really for Weight Loss?

There's a surprising amount of scientific research looking at the effectiveness of hypnosis of weight loss, and much of it is positive. One of the initial research carried out in 1986 showed that overweight women using a hypnosis system lost 17 pounds compared to 0.5 pounds for people just told to watch what they were eating. A meta-analysis of studies into hypnosis weight loss found in the 1990s that people who used hypnosis lost more than twice as much weight than those who did not.

And a study in 2014 showed that women who used hypnosis were enhancing their weight, BMI, eating habits, and even other aspects of body image.

Yet it's not just good news: A 2012 Stanford report found that about a fifth of people actually can not be hypnotized and it has nothing to do with their personalities, contrary to common opinion. Instead, the brains of some people just do not seem to work this way. "If you're not prone to daydreaming, you still find it hard to get lost in a book or sit through a movie and don't think you 're imaginative, you may be one of the people for whom hypnosis isn't working well," says Dr. Stein.

Georgia is one of the success stories, for sure. She claims it not only helped her lose the extra pounds but helped her hold them off as well. Six years later, she kept her weight loss happily, occasionally checking back in with her hypnotherapist when she needs a refresher.

Hypnotherapy risks.

Again, most people see hypnosis as safe. Adverse reactions are uncommon.

Potential hazards include:

- Headache
- Dizziness
- Drowsiness
- Anxiety
- Fear
- The creation of false memory

Those who have hallucinations or delusions should speak to their doctor before trying hypnotherapy. Also, hypnosis under the influence of drugs or alcohol should not be done on a person.

Additional tips on losing weight:

Here are some things you can do at home to help with your efforts to lose weight:

Move your body most weekdays. Seek to get either 150 minutes of moderate exercise (such as cycling, water aerobics, gardening) or 75 minutes of more intensive workouts (such as biking, swimming laps, hiking) every week.

Keep a log on food. Track how much you consume, what you consume, and whether you eat out of hunger or not. Doing so will allow you to recognize shifting habits, including snacking out of boredom.

Eat vegetables and fruit. Aim for five fruit and vegetable servings each day. To curb your appetite, you should also add more fiber to your diet — between 25 to 30 grams every day.

Drink 6 to 8 glasses of water a day... Hydrated helps to reduce overeating.

Fight off the temptation to miss meals. Eating all day helps keep your metabolism going strong.

Weight loss surgery has been known as a fast response to the epidemic of obesity, and it is not exactly the magic wand; many believe it is. This book discusses the ten key differences between Gastric Band Hypnosis and Weight Loss Surgery.

1. The problems that caused the weight gain are still there after weight loss surgery!

What if the reason someone placed in excess weight on several stones had more to do with depression, anxiety, a response to a break-up, or other psychological or emotional problems than it did with food or excessive eating? And if we disregard all the complications and hazards associated with weight loss operation, the operation would only affect the patient's stomach. The issues that led to weight gain in the first place will not be addressed.

Therefore I am so excited about weight loss surgery. It is like dealing with a weeping child by cutting their chords of speech or stitching up their ears. This stops a child from crying, but it doesn't fix why the child is crying in the first place. The reason I created HypnoSlimming comes down to our core philosophy: change your mind, change your body!

2. Hypnosis to the gastric band is better than weight loss surgery

I'll expand on some of the specific reasons for the rest of the book, but Gastric Band Hypnosis is a series of specific suggestions to the unconscious mind that affects the appetite and urge to eat large amounts of food. Weight loss surgery, on the other hand, is an operation that physically alters your stomach and you have three more common problems other than occasional complications with general anesthesia:

Infection that causes about 1 in 20 people's blood clots in the legs (deep vein thrombosis) or lungs (pulmonary embolism) – this affects approximately 1 in 100 people with internal bleeding.

3. Hypnosis of the gastric band is less costly than weight loss surgery

There are differences in weight loss surgery, and it can affect the costs depending on the particular treatment. There are two principal methods of surgery for weight loss.

Restrictive surgery operates by reducing stomach size and stopping digestion. A normal gastric can hold about three pints of food. The stomach can at first contain as little as an ounce after surgery, but this may later extend to 2 or 3 ounces. The lower the intestine, the fewer you can eat. The less you eat, the more you lose your weight.

Malabsorbent/restrictive surgical procedures change how you take food. They give you a smaller stomach, and even lose or bypass part of your digestive tract, making it harder for your body to consume calories.Physicians no longer conduct solely malabsorbent operations — also called intestinal bypasses — due to the side effects.

Four common types of weight-loss surgery are:

- Roux-en-Y gastric bypass
- Laparoscopic adjustable gastric banding
- Sleeve gastrectomy
- Duodenal switch with biliopancreatic diversion

Typical procedures would range from £ 4,000 to £9,000. Gastric band hypnosis is much easier, and will usually take only two to three sessions with a professional practitioner. However, the procedure can occur in one session or just by listening to the audio, depending on the patient's suggestibility. For our Gastric Band Hypnosis care costs, please see our Tariffs or Offers section.

4. Hypnosis of gastric band doesn't leave scars

The trauma of undergoing surgery can leave both emotional scars and physical scarring. Naturally, physical injuries may disappear with time, but any weight loss obtained as a result of surgery that limits the consumption of food can seem like a hollow victory. It's like a middle-aged woman who's proud to be celibate while wearing a chastity belt. Sure, there is medical science to help with weight loss, but major changes in how psychological therapy can help with weight loss have been made in the past 30 years. These are only three examples of Hypnosis, NLP and gastric band hypnosis.

5. Surgical weight loss can cause gallstones

After weight loss surgery, about 1 in 12 people develop gallstones, usually ten months after surgery. Gallstones are tiny stones that form in the gallbladder, usually made of cholesterol. Gallstones often do not cause any symptoms. When they get stuck in a duct (an opening or channel), however, they may irritate and inflame the gallbladder and cause symptoms such as a sudden, extreme pain in your abdomen (tummy), nausea and vomiting or jaundice. I also help patients live healthier lives alongside gastric band hypnosis, reducing the likelihood of problems such as gallstones.

6. Gastric band hypnosis is not susceptible to stomal stenosis

Complication in people with a gastric bypass is that a piece of food may block the hole (stoma) connecting their stomach pouch to their small intestine. This is known as stomal stenosis and is believed to be 20 percent of people with a gastric bypass in one-fifth yes. (The above picture is another form of stomach problem).

Persistent vomiting is the commonest symptom of stomal stenosis.

Stomal stenosis may be treated by directing a small flexible tube, called an endoscope, to the stoma site. To unblock the stoma, a balloon attached to the endoscope is inflated.

The easiest way to avoid stomach stenosis is always to break food into tiny chunks, thoroughly chew the chunks, and avoid drinking during meals. Read all on life following surgery to lose weight.

7. Gastric band operation can cause food intolerance

About 1 in 35 people with a gastric band develop a food allergy, often many years after their service.

When the body is unable to tolerate certain foods, such as red meat or green salad, food intolerance results in a variety of unpleasant symptoms, such as:

Nausea

Vomiting

The disease of gastroesophageal reflux

It's unclear why a food intolerance can grow after surgery. Avoiding foods that cause a reaction may improve symptoms in most situations, but if you have recurring symptoms associated with a variety of different foods, removing the band and replacing it with a gastric bypass might be appropriate. That's approaching a weight loss surgery issue with even more weight loss surgery. Gastric band hypnosis has no side effects on these. Health, happiness, self-confidence, and a personal sense of pride are typical side effects of Gastric Band Hypnosis.

8. Gastric band slippage can be achieved with surgery but not with hypnosis of the gastric band

Slippage of the gastric band or lap band is a condition affecting around 1 in 50 people with a gastric band.

As the name indicates, after overeating, the band falls out of place, while the band is already attached. Which means that the stomach pouch is getting larger than it should be. This may cause such symptoms as:

- heartburn
- nausea
- vomiting

Additional surgery would be needed to repair the band, which entails further risks associated with surgery and body damage. The worst-case scenario with Gastric Band Hypnosis is that you may slip into old habits a few weeks, months, or even years after the therapy. For a top-up session, it is very easy to confirm Gastric Band Hypnosis suggestions. It is about an hour of relaxation, constructive ideas for confidence, and a sense of hope when the session is over. It is an appealing choice for a procedure that may require even more surgery in the future.

9. The risk of death with weight loss surgery is genuine

Here is what the NHS says about weight loss surgery's chance of death:

No operation is healthy, and all surgical operations threaten death. But with new procedures, the outlook for weight loss surgery has significantly improved. The chance of death in hospital following weight loss surgery of some sort is around 1 in 1,000. (Lottery winning odds are 1 in 14 million, meaning you 're 14,000 times more likely to die from weight loss surgery than winning the lottery.)

Weight loss surgery complications which can lead to death include:

- a pulmonary embolism that causes serious breathing difficulties and then death
- internal bleeding
- infection
- heart attack
- stroke

Several risk factors that increase the risk of death during or shortly after weight loss surgery have been identified. Those are:

- Aged over 45 years
- Blood pressure higher
- Has a BMI of 50 or greater
- Male, since obese men are more likely to weigh than obese women
- Has a known risk factor for lung embolism

Known risk factors for an embolism in the lungs include:

- Have past blood clot history;
- Pulmonary hypertension-especially high blood pressure within your lungs
- Syndrome of obesity hypoventilation – if you have persistent breathing difficulties associated with obesity

The above risk factors can have a major impact on the risk of death to your person. Untreated obesity, especially morbid obesity, does, however, carry a significant risk of premature death itself.

I accept that being obese brings health risks, but with all the risks discussed above, the solution is real surgery.

Chapter 6: UNDERSTANDING WHAT INTERMITTENT FASTING AND WHY IT IS THE SECRET TO LONG HEALTHY LIFE

What is Fasting Intermittent, and Why Should You Do It?

Intermittent fasting is not a diet; it is a food pattern. It is a way to prepare your meals, so you get the most out of them. Intermittent fasting doesn't affect what you eat; when you eat, it does.

Why is it worth change while you're eating?

Okay, most importantly, without going on an insane diet or eating your calories down to nil, it is a perfect way to get lean. Most of the time, when you start intermittent fasting, you'll try to keep your calories the same. (Most people eat bigger meals in a shorter time frame.) However, intermittent fasting is a safe way to keep the muscle mass on when leaning.

For all that has been said, the main reason people try intermittent fasting is to lose weight. We 're going to think about how intermittent fasts in a moment contribute to fat loss.

Most significantly, IF is one of the easiest ways we have to take off bad weight while retaining healthy weight because it requires very little change in behaviour. It is a positive thing, as it means intermittent fasting falls into the category of "easy enough to do it, but significant enough to make a difference."

Intermittent fasting increases several cardiovascular health measures in animals and humans, including blood pressure; heart rate rest; cholesterol, triglycerides, glucose, and insulin levels of high density and low-density lipoprotein (HDL and LDL); and insulin resistance.

Intermittent fasting also decreases markers of systemic

inflammation and oxidative stress associated with atherosclerosis.

Analysis of electrocardiographic studies shows that intermittent fasting improves variability in the heart rate by enhancing parasympathetic tone in rats and humans.

The CALERIE (Comprehensive Long-Term Effects Assessment of Reducing Energy Intake) research found that a 12 per cent reduction in average calorie intake over two years improves many cardiovascular risk factors in non-obese people.

A multicenter study found that regular caloric restriction improves many cardiometabolic risk factors in non-obese humans.46-50 Also, six short-term trials involving overweight or obese adults found that intermittent fasting is as successful for weight loss as standard diets.51 Two recent research showed that daily caloric restriction or intermittent fasting of 4:3 (24-hour three-time fasting)

However, in a 12-month study comparing alternate-day fasting, daily calorie restriction, and a placebo diet, participants in both intervention groups lost weight. Still, they had no changes in insulin sensitivity, lipid levels, or blood pressure as compared to control group participants.

Animal experiments indicate that intermittent fasting improves cognition in several areas, including spatial memory, associative memory, and working memory; alternate-day fasting and ordinary caloric restriction reverse spatial learning and adverse memory effects of obesity, diabetes, and neuroinflammation

Older adults on a short term caloric restriction diet had enhanced verbal memory in a clinical trial.

A research involving overweight adults with mild cognitive impairment led to improvements in verbal memory, executive function, and global cognition for 12 months of caloric restriction. More recently, a massive, multicenter, randomized clinical trial found that two years of daily caloric restriction led to a substantial improvement in working memory. Additional studies of intermittent fasting and cognition in older people need to be conducted, especially given the absence of any pharmacological therapies that influence brain ageing and neurodegenerative progression

Intermittent fasting clinical trials in cancer patients have been completed, or are ongoing. Many of the initial research concentrated on biomarker enforcement, side effects and characterization. A routine caloric restriction check in men with prostate cancer, for example, demonstrated excellent adherence (95 per cent) with no adverse effects. Several case studies involving glioblastoma patients indicate intermittent fasting can suppress tumour growth and prolong survival.

Intermittent-fasting regimens minimize tissue damage and enhance the functional outcomes in animal models of traumatic and ischemic tissue injury.

Preoperative fasting prevents tissue damage and inflammation, which increases the outcomes of surgery. In animal models of vascular surgical damage, ischemia-reperfusion cost in the liver and kidneys was decreased by three days of fasting, and intimate hyperplasia in trauma-induced carotid-artery was reduced before the injury. A randomized, multicenter study found that two weeks of daily preoperative energy restriction improves outcomes in patients undergoing gastric bypass surgery. Such results indicate that intermittent preoperative fasting can be a safe and efficient way to improve surgical outcomes.

Professionals like dietitians, exercise physiologists and psychologists can help to boost your motivation and knowledge to help you achieve your goals for weight loss.

Declining weight decreases asthma symptoms in obese patients. In one trial, patients adhering to the alternate-day fasting regimen had an elevated serum level of ketone bodies on energy-restriction days. They lost weight over a 2-month period over which symptoms of asthma and resistance to airways were mitigated. A reduction in symptoms has been associated with significant decreases in serum levels of inflammation and oxidative stress markers.

Multiple sclerosis is an inflammatory disease of the central nervous system characterized by demyelination of the axon and neuronal degeneration. In a rat model of multiple sclerosis (experimentally induced autoimmune encephalomyelitis), alternate-day fasting and intermittent periods of 3 consecutive days of energy restriction minimize autoimmune demyelination and boost the functional outcome.

HOW INTERMITTENT FASTING WORKS

We need to comprehend the difference between the fed state and the fasted state to understand how intermittent fasting contributes to fat loss.

As it digests and absorbs food, the body is in a fed state. Usually, after you start eating the fed state starts and lasts three to five hours while your body absorbs and digest the food you just ate. It is very difficult for your body to burn fat while you are in the fed state since your insulin levels are high.

After that period, your body goes into what is called the post-absorptive state, which is just a fancy way of saying your body is not eating a meal.

The post – the absorptive cycle lasts up to 8 to 12 hours after your last meal, which is when you hit the fasted time limit. Burning fat is much healthier for your body in the fasted state since your insulin levels are low.

If you're in a fasted state, your body will burn inaccessible fat during the fed state.

Since we are not entering the fasted state until 12 hours after our last meal, it is unusual for our bodies to be in this state of fat burning. That is one of the reasons that many people who begin intermittent fasting lose weight without adjusting what they eat, how often they sleep, or how much they exercise.

Fasting brings your body to a state of fat burning, which you rarely do during a normal eating schedule.

THE INTERMITTENT FASTING HISTORY

Intermittent fasting is perhaps the oldest known dieting method. It dates back to the onset of human history.

For centuries IF has not only been actively practiced by Greek philosophers and Eastern mystics but also IF has existed naturally throughout human history. Hunter-gatherers had a much more difficult time getting three meals a day. Therefore the human body has evolved to be able to survive long periods without food and even expect them to.

It is a fairly new development compared to the period of human existence – the refrigerator and the grocery store, which enables the average human being to consume whatever, whenever. Such quick access to food has resulted in compulsive, pleasure-seeking eating that contributes to obesity and has eliminated fasting 's normal occurrence. This event provides several benefits for our bodies.

Fortunately, intermittent fasting is beginning to grow in popularity, and many modern-day medical studies have only further demonstrated the ancient beliefs about the benefits of fasting.

'Fasting intermittent' Diet could improve your health

"The state of the science on IF has evolved to the point that it can now be seen as one approach to improving and maintaining health as a lifestyle approach, with exercise and healthy food," said senior author Mark Mattson, a neuroscientist with Johns Hopkins Medicine in Baltimore.

There are two key ways to fasten your life intermittently, Mattson said:

- Daily, time-limited feeding offers you a small window to eat, usually 6-8 hours a day.
- 5:2 Intermittent fasting allows people to eat just one moderate-sized meal every two days.

When people fast, they burn slowly through the glucose stored in their liver, explained Mattson. The liver has a glucose content of about 700 calories.

"Taking up the energy reserves of the liver takes 10 to 12 hours," Mattson said. "What happens then is that the fats are used for energy."

This cycle is called "metabolic switching," and American-favoured three-meal-a-day eating pattern doesn't allow their bodies to run through the energy reserves of their liver and make the turn to fat burning, Mattson said.

In the new paper, the latest empirical evidence was presented by Mattson and colleagues. Studies show sporadic fasts may be:

- Regulate blood sugar levels, improve stress tolerance, and cushion inflammation.
- Reduce blood pressure and cholesterol, and increase heart rate.
- Improve memory and brain health.

"If you're thinking of IF as a fad diet, I think it's a relatively valid choice," said Hannah Kittrell, a registered dietitian and manager of the New York City Mount Sinai PhysioLab, a nutrition and physiology exercise clinic.

"The reason is it doesn't cut out any food groups completely," said Kittrell, who wasn't part of the study. "It's not that you don't eat sugar, you don't eat fat, it just modulates when you eat food."

Kittrell said her lab measures various diets by looking at their social, historical, and biological background, and all three assessments pass intermittent fasting.

"There is an evolutionary justification in the sense that hunter-gatherers adopted an intermittent fasting diet because the food was scarce. The next time they were eating, they would not learn," she said.

The Mattson-described metabolic transition represents the biological basis of intermittent fasting, and history is full of examples of fasting humans, Kittrell said.

"For religious and medical cal purposes it has been used a great deal," Kittrell said. "Ramadan is an outstanding example of prolonged intermittent fasting."

Mattson sets out a variety of sample prescriptions in the paper to integrate fasting into your everyday life.

Individuals who want to try time-limited feeding may restrict themselves for the first month to a 10-hour feeding period five days a week, then drop the duration down to eight and then six hours in subsequent months. The target would be to get seven days a week to 6-hour feeding time, the researchers wrote.

Or people could start by fasting one day a week, with one meal on that 1,000-calorie day, and by the second month extending it to two days a week. A single 500-calorie meal will be the target for two days per week.

Mattson and Kittrell say you will possibly find yourself anxious as your body adapts to your new eating style.

"This is likewise similar to exercise programs where a sedentary person takes a couple of months to get in shape while their organ systems adapt to the exercise,"

It can take someone to get comfortable with intermittent fasting from a few weeks and a couple of months, Mattson and Kittrell said.

"If someone normally eats breakfast, and they don't eat breakfast tomorrow, they'll be hungry and irritable when it gets to lunchtime," Mattson said. "If they stick with it, it will be gone after two weeks to a month. This is a very significant practical thing."

Neither expects immediate results — it can take a few weeks before the body adapts to the point where you start falling pounds and having improved measures of health, Mattson said.

Participants must also note that fasting does not grant them free license to eat whatever they want, Kittrell said.

"You do want to have a balanced diet," Kittrell said. "It's not like you can just eat fast food, but you're going to be safe when you're doing intermittent fasting."

Though Kittrell finds intermittent fasting to be a good diet choice, she said there is still much to learn about it.

Studies, for example, show that some people respond better than others to fasting, although she said the reasons why they are not yet understood.

"I think it's exciting, but there's still a lot of work to do before you can claim intermittent fasting is 100 % safe and successful for all to adopt," said Kittrell.

Mattson, who has been fasting himself for 20 years, said that there are some groups of people he wouldn't advocate the practice for — youth, the elderly and people who already have very low body weight.

He agrees with Kittrell that more work is needed on the potential of fasting for safety.

For one thing, there is a good case to make that intermittent fasting might strengthen the cancer treatment, Mattson said.

"It turns out that cancer cells typically only use glucose as a food source," Mattson said. "They can not use fats. "If the person is fasting, if you strike them with chemotherapeutic drugs or radiation, then their cancer cells are easier to kill."

Multiple trials are still underway to see whether fasting will help cure cancer, Mattson noted.

10 EVIDENCE-BASED PROLONGED FASTING HEALTH BENEFITS

1. Intermittent changes in fasting The function of cells, genes, and hormones

Several things happen in your body when you are not feeding for a while.

For example, your body begins important processes of cellular repair and adjusts the hormone levels, so that stored body fat becomes more available.

Here are some of the changes that occur during fasting in your body:

- Insulin levels: Insulin levels drop dramatically in the blood, promoting fat burning.
- Human growth hormone: growth hormone blood levels can increase up to 5-fold. Higher levels of this hormone promote burning fat and building muscle and have several other benefits.

- Cellular repair: The body causes essential processes of cellular repairs, such as removing waste material from cells.
- Gene expression: Different genes and molecules have beneficial effects related to survival and disease prevention.

These changes in hormones, gene expression and cell function are related to many of the benefits of intermittent fasting.

When you are fast, the insulin levels drop, and the hormone of human growth rises. Also, your cells initiate essential processes of cellular repair and alter through genes they express.

2. Fasting intermittent will help you lose weight and belly fat

Many of those who try intermittent fasting do so for weight loss. The intermittent fasting would usually help you eat fewer meals. If you make up for that by eating even more during the other meals, you will end up consuming fewer calories.

Furthermore, intermittent fasting improves hormone activity to prevent weight loss.

Lower levels of insulin, higher levels of growth hormone, and elevated concentrations of norepinephrine (noradrenaline) all increase body fat breakdown and promote its energy usage. Short-term fasting raises your metabolic rate by 3.6-14 per cent, which lets you consume even more calories.

Intermittent fasting, in other words, operates on both sides of the calorie equation. This increases your metabolic rate and reduces the amount of food you consume (reduces calories in). Intermittent fasting can cause weight loss of 3-8 per cent over 3-24 weeks, according to a 2014 analysis of the scientific literature. This is an incredible number.

People have lost 4-7 per cent of their waist circumference, meaning they lost tons of belly fat, the unhealthy fat that causes disease in the abdominal cavity. One research study also found that intermittent fasting resulted in less muscle loss than a constant limit on calories.

IF helps you eat fewer calories, while slightly improving your metabolism. It's a very powerful tool for weight loss and stomach fat loss.

3. Intermittent fasting will reduce resistance to insulin, lower the risk of type 2 diabetes

Over recent times, type 2 diabetes has become extremely prevalent. Its key characteristic in terms of insulin resistance is elevated blood sugar levels. Anything that increases resistance to insulin will help reduce blood sugar levels and protect against type 2 diabetes.

Ironically, intermittent fasting has been shown to have important benefits for insulin resistance, contributing to a remarkable drop in blood sugar.

Fasting blood sugar has been reduced by 3-6% in human experiments on intermittent fasting while fasting insulin has been reduced by 20-31%. Only one study in diabetic rats found that intermittent fasting protected against kidney damage, one of the most serious diabetes complications.

What this implies is that intermittent fasting for people at risk of developing type 2 diabetes can be highly protective.

There can be some differences between genders, however. One female research found that blood sugar regulation gradually decreased after an intermittent fasting regimen that lasted for 22 days.

Intermittent fasting, at least in people, can reduce insulin resistance and lower blood sugar levels.

4. Intermittent fasting can reduce oxidative stress and body inflammation

One of the steps towards ageing and other chronic diseases is oxidative stress. It involves unstable molecules, named free radicals, which react to and damage other essential molecules (such as protein and DNA). Several research shows that intermittent fasting can enhance the body's oxidative stress resistance.

Additionally, studies show intermittent fasting can help combat inflammation, another main cause of chronic diseases of all kinds.

Studies show that intermittent fasting is capable of reducing body oxidative damage and inflammation. It would have advantages against ageing and multiple diseases emerging.

5. Fasting intermittent can be beneficial for heart health

Heart disease is the greatest killer in the world right now.

It is understood that specific health markers (so-called "risk factors") are either associated with an increased or reduced risk of heart disease. Numerous specific risk factors like blood pressure, total and LDL cholesterol, blood triglycerides, inflammatory markers and blood sugar levels have been shown to boost intermittent fasting. Most of this is, however, focused on animal research. There is a need to study the impact on heart safety even more in humans before recommendations can be made.

Studies show that intermittent fasting can enhance various heart disease risk factors such as blood pressure, cholesterol levels, triglycerides and inflammatory markers.

6. Intermittent fasting causes different mechanisms of cellular repair

The cells in the body initiate a process of cellular "waste removal" called autophagy when we fast. It includes breaking down the cells and metabolizing the damaged and defective proteins that over time build up within the cells. Enhanced autophagy may protect against a variety of illnesses, including cancer and Alzheimer's.

Fasting activates a metabolic path called autophagy which removes cells from waste material.

7. Intermittent fasting help prevent cancer

Cancer is a horrible disease which is characterized by uncontrolled cell growth. Fasting has been shown to have some beneficial effects on metabolism, which may contribute to reduced cancer risk.

Despite the need for human studies, promising evidence from animal studies suggests that intermittent fasting may help to prevent cancer. There is also some evidence for patients with human cancer which indicates that fasting has reduced various side effects of chemotherapy. In animal, studies it has been shown that intermittent fasting helps to prevent cancer. One paper in humans has shown that chemotherapy can reduce side effects.

8. intermittent fasting is healthy for the brain

Also, what is good for the body is good for the brain too.

Intermittent fasting strengthens the different metabolic features that are considered to be critical for brain health. This includes reduced oxidative stress, decreased inflammation and decreased levels of blood sugar and insulin resistance.

Several rat studies have shown that intermittent fasting can stimulate the development of new nerve cells, which would improve brain function. This also raises brain hormone levels called brain-derived neurotrophic factor (BDNF), a deficit affecting depression and many other brain issues.

Animal tests have also shown that prolonged fasting by stroke protects against brain damage. Intermittent fasting will bring important benefits for the health of the brain. It can increase neuronal growth and protect the brain against damage.

9. Fasting intermittent Can help prevent Alzheimer's disease

Alzheimer's disease is on the most common neurodegenerative condition in the world.

There is no treatment available for Alzheimer's, and it is important to keep it from occurring in the first place.

A rat study shows intermittent fasting can postpone the onset of Alzheimer's disease or decrease its severity. A lifestyle change that involved regular short-term fasts could dramatically boost Alzheimer's symptoms in 9 out of 10 patients in a series of case reports. Animal studies also show that fasting will protect against other neurodegenerative disorders, including disease caused by Parkinson and Huntington. There is, therefore, a need for further human research.

Animal studies show intermittent fasting may be protective against neurodegenerative disorders such as Alzheimer's disease.

10. Fasting intermittent can prolong your life, allow you to live longer

Some of the intermittent fasting's most promising uses may be its potential to prolong lifespan.

Research in rats has shown that intermittent fasting similarly increases lifespan to constant restriction of calories.

The effects had been quite dramatic in some of these studies. For one of them, rats who fasted every other day lived 83 per cent longer than non-fasted rats. While this is far from being proved in humans, intermittent fasting among the anti-ageing crowd has become very common. Given the known metabolism benefits and all sorts of health markers, it makes sense that intermittent fasting might help you live longer, healthier lives.

THE BENEFITS OF INTERMITTENT FASTING

Fat loss is fantastic, but fasting is not the only benefit.

1. Intermittent fasts simplify your day.

I 'm focused on improvement in attitude, consistency and stress management. Intermittent fasting gives my life extra simplicity which I enjoy. I don't think about breakfast when I wake up. I just grab a glass of water and get my day started.

I love eating, and I don't mind cooking, so eating three meals a day has never been a trouble for me. Intermittent fasting, however, helps me to eat one less meal, which also means to prepare one less meal, cook one less meal and think over one less meal. It makes life a little easier, and that is what I want.

2. Continuous fasting lets you live longer.

For a while, scientists have understood that reducing calories is a way of prolonging life. From a logical perspective, this makes sense. Your body finds ways of extending your life when you're hungry.

There is only one issue: Who wants to eat for longer in the name of living?

I don't know about you, but I do want to live a long life. Hunger for myself, does not sound so appealing.

The good news is that intermittent fasting stimulates many of the same life-extending mechanisms as calorie restricting. In other words, without the hassle of starvation, you get the rewards of a longer life.

3. Intermittent fasting can reduce cancer risk.

That one is up for discussion since not much work and testing has been conducted on the cancer-fasting relationships. Nonetheless, early signs do look promising.

This study of 10 cancer patients indicates that before diagnosis, the side effects of chemotherapy can be reduced by fasting. This RESULT finding is also confirmed by another study that used alternate day fasting for cancer patients and concluded that it would result in better cure rates and fewer deaths before chemotherapy.

Finally, this systematic review of multiple fasting and disease research has concluded that fasting not only tends to reduce cancer risk but also cardiovascular disease.

4. Intermittent fasting is considerably better than dieting.

It's not because we switch to the wrong foods that most diets fail; it's because we don't follow the diet over the long run. This is not a question of diet; it is a question of a change in behaviour.

That is where intermittent fasting shines because when you get past the notion that you ought to eat all the time, it's surprisingly easy to enforce. For instance, this study found intermittent fasting to be an effective weight-loss strategy for obese adults and concluded that "subjects adapt quickly" to an IF routine.

I like the quote below from Dr Michael Eades, who tried to fast himself intermittently, about the difference between attempting a diet and attempting intermittent fasting.

"Diets are easy to contemplate and hard to execute. Intermittent fasting is just the opposite — in contemplation it's difficult, but in execution, it's simple.

Some of us have been considering going on a diet. Once we come across a diet that appeals to us, it seems like it's going to be a breeze to do. Yet it gets tough when we get into the nitty-gritty of it. For starters, I stay almost all the time on a low-carb diet. But if I think a low-fat diet is going on, it looks simple. I 'm referring to bagels, whole wheat bread and jam, mashed potatoes, peas, twelve bananas, etc.—all of which sound appealing. But if I were to embark on such a low-fat diet, I would soon be sick of it and want meat and eggs to be available. So in reflection, a diet is easy, but not so easy in practice in the long term.

In reflection, intermittent fasting is hard, about which there is no doubt. "You walk 24 hours without food? "When we explained what we were doing, people would ask, incredulously. "I will never be able to do that." But it's a snap once started. No questions about when and where one or two of the three meals a day will be consumed. This is a perfect deliverance. Expenditure on your food is plummeting. And you're not particularly hungry. ... Even though it's hard to conquer the thought of going without food, nothing could be simpler once you start the routine.

— Dr Michael Eades

The simplicity of intermittent fasting is, in my opinion, the biggest reason to give it a try. This offers a wide variety of health benefits without seeking a drastic change in lifestyle.

Benefits

The most noticeable advantage of intermittent fasting is weight loss.

There are also other advantages beyond this, some of which have been recognized since ancient times.

The fasting cycles have also been called 'cleanses,' 'detoxifications' or 'purifications,' but the concept is similar – to abstain for a certain amount of time from consuming food. People assumed that this duration of food abstinence would kill and rejuvenate their toxin systems.

Some of the intermittent fasting 's alleged health benefits include:

- A lack of weight and body fat
- Benefit in fat burning
- Reduced insulin and sugar levels in the blood
- Reversal possible Type 2 diabetes
- Mental focus and attention probably improved
- Potential energy boost
- Possible growth hormone increase, at least in the short term
- Probably higher cholesterol in the blood
- Possibly longer life
- Activation of cellular cleaning possible by inducing autophagy
- Potentially reduced inflammation

Fasting also provides other significant special benefits that aren't present in traditional diets.

While diets can complicate life, it can be simplified with intermittent fasting. While diets can take time, it saves time to fast. While diets may be restricted in variety, fasting is available wherever possible.

To lose weight

Intermittent fasting at its very heart helps the body to use its stored energy effectively by burning off excess body fat.

It is important to remember that this is natural and that humans have evolved to fast for shorter periods of time-hours or days-without adverse health effects.

Body fat is merely energy extracted away from the food. If you're not eating, your body just "eats" its fat for energy.

Life is about equilibrium—the poor and the strong, the yin and the yang. The same holds for feeding and fasting. After all, fasting is the flip side of food. If you don't feed, then you fast.

Here's how things work:

When we eat, it ingests more food energy than can be used immediately. To later usage, some of the energy needs to be put away. Insulin is the main hormone involved in food energy storage.

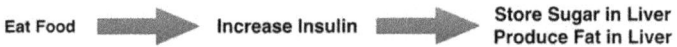

Eat Food ➡ Increase Insulin ➡ **Store Sugar in Liver**
Produce Fat in Liver

When we eat insulin increases, helping to store the extra sugar in two distinct ways. Carbohydrates are broken down into individual units of glucose (sugar), which can be linked into long chains to form glycogen, and then stored in the liver or muscle.

However, there is very little storage space for carbohydrates; and once that is reached, the liver begins to convert the excess glucose into fat. This process is termed de-novo lipogenesis (which means "making new fat").

Most of these newly produced fat will be retained in the liver, but much of it will be transferred to other body fat deposits. Although this method is more complex, there is virtually no limit to the amount of fat that can be produced.

Therefore, our bodies have two complementary mechanisms for storing food resources. One is readily available but has minimal storage space (glycogen), and the other is more difficult to access but has nearly infinite storage space (body fat).

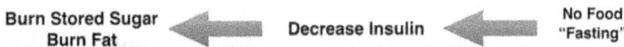

Burn Stored Sugar ⬅ Decrease Insulin ⬅ **No Food**
Burn Fat **"Fasting"**

When we don't eat, the process goes in reverse. Insulin levels are decreasing, causing the body to start consuming stored energy as no more food comes in.

Slow start. Das recommends undertaking a week of intermittent fasting and seeing how you're doing. There are various forms of intermittent fasting — from the time-limited diet, which restricts diet to a specific time-window (such as noon to 8:00 pm), to rotating day fasting, which includes fasting every other day. Find what's right for you. "Time-bound fasting makes the most natural diet patterns," Cox says, which could make it more doable. Instead of eating just a few hundred calories or cutting off food altogether during periods of fasting, "start by limiting your calorie intake to only half or 75% of your normal calorie intake," Pan says. "Scale-up then."

You may be overeating.

"Non-fasting days are not days where you can splurge absolutely," Das says. Otherwise, you may end up with a net calorie surplus which leads to weight gain. Once again, the challenge is that fasting can potentially cause binge eating. In a five-year study of 496 teenage girls, binge-eating was strongly predicted by the fasting — which the researchers described as not eating for a 24-hour weight control span. Additionally, a 2015 study showed that fasting dramatically increased stress hormone cortisol levels, which can lead to cravings. It does make sense.

"If you're used to eating three meals ... maybe a snack in between, it's a big change when you're doing intermittent fasting," Pan says. "That can cause some people to experience increased stress levels."

If you're a stress eater, try cortisol-lowering behaviours such as meditating or listening to music. Recall even filling up healthy, satiating foods during feeding times.

You may become dehydrated.

"Intermittent fasting is sometimes associated with dehydration, because you may forget to drink when you don't eat," says Pan. Need to pay careful attention to the thirsty signs of your body during times of fasting.

You may feel tired.

Feeling groggy is common, particularly as an intermittent, fasting newbie. Your body runs on less energy than normal, and because fasting can increase stress rates, it can also interfere with your sleep habits, Pan says. Seek meditating or other behaviours that reduce tension. When you have a daily exercise routine, schedule your workouts during times of feeding, Cox says. It would not only help you save energy but exercising while fasting may lead to low levels of blood sugar, the symptoms of which – such as dizziness and discomfort – may increase the risk of injury.

You may be feeling irritable.

"The same biochemistry that controls mood also controls appetite," says Steiger, with nutrient intake influencing neurotransmitter activity such as dopamine and serotonin, which play a role in anxiety and depression. Which means your appetite dysregulation will do the same to your mood. Stick to a nutritionally balanced, satiating diet during your eating periods again and remember to clock in enough sleep, which research has also linked to mood.

You could get drunk a lot easier

It's ok to imbibe during intermittent fasting but after fasting periods not during or immediately. As you probably have found out firsthand, if you drink on an empty stomach, you can get drunker faster.

That said, even if you restrict your drinking to eating hours, "you displace the potential for proper nutrition"—which already restricts intermittent fasting—"with alcohol," says Cox. So if weight loss is the objective, low-nutrient, high-calorie alcohol "is not our best option."

We may not know the long-term consequences. Of course,

intermittent fasting studies so far show that it will help you lose weight for a few months — but we don't have the long-term evidence to decide whether you're going to be able to hold it off years later, or whether sustained intermittent fasting is even safe or healthy, Cox says. She advises anyone who considers intermittent fasting to speak to their doctor, but "particularly if they want to do it on a long-term basis to make sure this is their best choice."

10 FASTING SIDE EFFECTS THAT THAT COULD MEAN IT IS NOT A GOOD IDEA FOR YOU

Intermittent fasting (IF) fans are positively raving about all the potential benefits, indeed. But behind all the talk about what kind of fasting schedule is right for you, or whether you can combine IF with other diets like keto, there is a frequently overlooked fact: Intermittent Fasting can still cause side effects or have its negative effects ... especially if you don't do it right.

"It 's important to find out the type of IF works for you, whether it's a shorter or longer fasting period or only doing it so many days a week," says Alyssa Koens, head of weight loss coaching company Profile Sanford, a registered dietitian.

"When you eat too few calories or nutrients during periods of fasting, you may have side effects."

But since there are no formal guidelines on how many calories you should be consuming during IF — or what kinds of foods you should be filling on during non-fasting hours — it can be difficult to hit you IF groove without first hitting some bumps on the road ... assuming it's even the right decision for you. And there are some signs to watch out for that may mean it's simply not the best fit for you and your lifestyle.

But first: If you're wondering why It is so common in the first place, intermittent fasting may have potential benefits.

There are some possible beneficial benefits of IF including weight loss, greater regulation of appetite and lower levels of insulin. The key concern is that none of those benefits has in any way been thoroughly investigated. The research is also the most sparse in humans (compared to, say, mice studies).

It is also unclear whether the root cause of the alleged benefits is intermittent self-fasting (e.g. how it affects your body, say, at a cellular level) or just calorie restriction.

So at this point, it is kind of a trial and error to see if an Intermittent Fasting eating style works for you and your body.

On the other hand, several potential negative side effects with IF are present.

The upsides of intermittent fasting, as described, are still very much in the research process, but there are some encouraging findings there. There is also plenty of anecdotal evidence, however, that IF comes with some potentially negative side effects, so you shouldn't initiate an IF eating program without first working out certain issues with your doctor.

Here are ten red flags to watch out for. So if you experience any of these side effects before continuing, this means stopping IF and talking to your doctor or nutritionist.

1. Feel hungry

We 're not 100 per cent sure "hangriness" is a real term, but it's certainly a real feeling. That's the feeling of grouchiness, grumpiness, or overall irritability that comes with being unable to eat when your body tells you it's hungry.

As previously stated by WH, preparing the body to go 16 hours without food requires some practice, even within a limited timeframe, the bodies of certain people may not ever be comfortable eating.

In principle, you shouldn't be hungry first thing in the morning if you are eating enough protein later in the day or night. So if you are, this is an indication that during your caloric intake cycle you need to make some dietary changes to stop transforming into a big crank — or it's an indication that you're just not vibrating well with fasting. With certain people (e.g. those who work out a ton), it might just not be suitable for them to eat for long periods — and that's certainly something worth considering. Don't force them.

2. Fatigue or brain fog

Have you ever found yourself gaining over and over the middle of the morning, only to realize that you have never had breakfast before? Because not consuming breakfast is usually the way most people do IF, noticing that you're overly exhausted every day — or making stupid mistakes because you're wading through brain fog — is a tip-off that you don't eat the right food during non-fasting hours, or that fasting doesn't suit your lifestyle requirements.

"Watch out what you're feeding your body with," Koens says. " Whether you can eat what you want, but you should always be fueling it with good food that will make you feel safe and solid." And if you're just feeling * way * better breakfast most days, listen to your body.

3. Being fascinated with food

Going on any sort of restrictive diet will impact your food relationship, Koens says. Although some people like IF 's rigidity, others might be more focused on when they should eat, and how many calories they get.

Spending too much time thinking about the quality or quantity of your daily food can lead to a certain type of eating disorder called orthorexia. According to The National Association of Eating Disorders, having orthorexia means that you focus so much on "right" or "good" eating that it hurts your overall wellbeing.

This should not be the goal of any diet. Koens says: "You want to concentrate on developing a safe, meaningful food relationship."

4. Blood sugar lower

During IF, if you're experiencing constant nausea, headaches, or dizziness, that's a red flag suggesting the diet may throw your blood sugar out of whack. As previously stated by WH, diabetics should for this very reason avoid any form of fasting diet: IF may cause you to become hypoglycemic, a dangerous condition for anyone with insulin or thyroid problems.

5. Loss of hair

Seriously, then? Yup ...... yup. Koens says that sudden weight loss or lack of adequate nutrients, especially protein and B vitamins, can lead to hair loss.

A significant point: while IF doesn't automatically lead to a nutrient loss, consuming a well-rounded diet appears to be harder when you cram a whole day of consuming in a few hours. If you find more hair is falling out every day in the shower than normal, re-evaluate the nutritional quality of your regular meals and speak to your doctor about whether This is a good step for you.

6. Changes in your menstrual cycle

Here's a side effect of quick weight loss (which can be attributed to IF): women who lose a dramatic amount of weight or who regularly don't get enough calories every day can find their menstrual cycles slowing down or even stopping altogether.

People that have unusually low body weight are vulnerable to a disorder called amenorrhea, or lack of menstruation, per the Mayo Clinic. Sudden weight loss or underweight can interfere with your normal hormone cycle and cause missed periods; so while you may be pleased about how It has helped you lose pounds, you may also deprive your body of the calories it requires to work.

Stop fasting and speak to your gynaecologist about troubleshooting if you miss having your period and suspect it's due to intermittent fasting practices you 're practising.

7. Constipation

All got backed up? IF may be guilty. "Any diet can cause stomach upset if you don't get enough food, vitamins, protein or fibre," says Koens, who stresses the importance of keeping hydrated during the day.

It's easy for people to forget to drink water during fasting hours, she says, but going 16 hours a day without adequate fluid is a recipe for a (gastrointestinal) catastrophe.

And if you've begun an IF diet and you don't seem to be able to get your bowel movements to happen consistently (or at all), it's time to pause on your program and talk to a nutritionist or doctor about what's going on (in this case, or not!).

8. Unhealthy diet

Even though It does not cause severe illness such as orthorexia, it may also lead to some pretty poor eating behaviours. Besides not having the necessary nutrients, during non-fasting hours, you may also find yourself making messy, unhealthy choices.

"The biggest problem is setting off binge-eating behaviour, when you're so hungry that you're consuming 5,000 calories [and going well over your normal amount]," Charlie Seltzer, MD, weight-loss physician and licensed personal trainer told WH before.

If that sounds like you, you may be better off working with an RD to find a strategy that doesn't push you to limit your eating hours and instead focuses on feeding your body with the right nutrients around the clock, not in a particular window.

9.Sleep disorders

Koens says that many people show better sleep patterns when doing IF, probably because of how IF helps curb late-night snacking behaviours, and in effect, an inability to fall asleep because your stomach is still busy digesting that at 10 pm. Yeah, nosh.

Some work does point to the opposite effect, though. A 2018 study in the journal Nature and Science of Sleep provides evidence that intermittent diurnal fasting (meaning daytime fasting) induces a drop in rapid-eye sleep (REM) movement. According to the Harvard Business Review, getting enough REM sleep was linked to all sorts of health benefits, including cognitive processing, better memory, and concentration.

It's unclear exactly why.

If you find that after you have begun an IF eating program, you can't fall asleep or stay asleep again, press pause and speak to a pro to make sure you don't harm your wellbeing.

10. Change in mood

This would be odd if, at least at the beginning, you were not feeling any moodiness or * ahem * hangry during IF. And while some people experience a big boost in energy or motivation once they transition to fasting, it's important to note that it's still a restrictive diet. Feeling compelled to obey it could have negative effects on your mood, particularly if you are becoming isolated from family members or friends due to restrictions on your diet.

If you're feeling down, nervous, or depressed about It, stopping and getting in contact with a licensed dietitian, counsellor, or wellness coach immediately is key. They could help you build a fasting schedule that fits your mind and body better.

Chapter 7: FASTING AND AUTOPHAGY

But what exactly is autophagy? The Greek term derives from auto (self) and phagein (eat). Therefore the term means eating yourself. Essentially, this is the body's mechanism to get rid of all the broken down, old cell machinery (organelles, proteins, and cell membranes) when there is not enough energy to sustain it any longer. The degradation and recycling of cellular components are controlled orderly process.

There is a similar, better-known process, also known as programmed cell death called apoptosis. Cells are made to die after a certain number of divisions. Although this may at first sound like horrible, remember that this phase is key to preserving good health. Suppose you possess a vehicle, for example. You love the car. You've got big memories in it.

But it starts looking sort of beat-up after a few years. It doesn't look so great, after a few more. The vehicle costs you thousands of dollars for repairs each year. The entire time, it breaks down. Is it easier to keep that around because it's just a hunk of junk? Of course not. So, you 're getting rid of it and buying an excellent new car.

The same is evident in the body. Cells are getting old and junky. It's easier to have them programmed to die when their useful lives are finished. It sounds cruel, but it's life. That is the apoptosis process, where cells are predestined to die after some time. This is like leasing a vehicle. You get rid of the car after a certain amount of time, whether it is still going or not. Then you get yourself a new car. You should not think about breaking things down at the worst possible moment.

Autophagy-replacing old cell parts

On a subcellular level, too, the same process happens. You don't have to replace the whole car, necessarily. You just have to replace the battery sometimes, throw the old one out and get a new one. It occurs in the cells, too. Rather of destroying the whole cell (apoptosis), you just want to destroy certain pieces of the cell. That is the autophagy process, where subcellular organelles are destroyed, and new ones are rebuilt to replace them. You can remove old membranes, organelles, and other cellular debris. It is achieved by sending it to the lysosome that is a complex organelle that produces protein degrading enzymes.

Autophagy was first explained in 1962 when researchers observed an increase in the number of lysosomes in rat liver cells after infusing glucagon (the part of the cell that destroys stuff). Nobel laureate scientist Christian de Duve coined the term autophagy. Damaged subcellular sections and unused proteins are marked for destruction and then sent to the lysosomes for completion of the work.

One of the main autophagy regulators is kinase known as rapamycin (mTOR) mammalian target. It suppresses autophagy when mTOR is activated and promotes it when dormant.

What Triggers Autophagy?

Deprivation of nutrients is the main activator of autophagy. Recall that insulin is kind of the opposite hormone to glucagon. It's like the game that we played as children - 'opposite day.' When insulin goes up, then glucagon will go down. When insulin goes down, then glucagon will go up. The insulin goes up when we chew, and the glucagon goes down. When we don't eat (fast), insulin will go down, and glucagon will go up. The glucagon increase stimulates the autophagy cycle. Fasting (raises glucagon) potentially gives the biggest known boost to autophagy.

Fasting is also much more effective than merely inducing autophagy. They 're doing two good things.

We 're cleaning out all our old, junky proteins and cellular pieces by inducing autophagy. Simultaneously, fasting also stimulates growth hormone, which tells our body to start producing some new attractive body parts. We are giving the whole renovation to our bodies.

You need to get rid of the old stuff before you can bring new stuff in. Think about getting your kitchen renovated. If you have old lime green cabinets sitting around in the 1970s era, you need to junk them before you bring some new ones in. Therefore, the destruction process (removal) is just as critical as the creation process. If you were simply trying to bring the old cabinets in without taking them out, it wouldn't look so bright. So fasting may reverse the ageing process in some ways, by getting rid of old cellular junk and replacing it with new pieces.

A highly regulated mechanism

Autophagy is a process which has strong regulations. This would be harmful if it runs amok out of sight, so it must be carefully managed. Total loss of amino acids in mammalian cells is a strong signal for autophagy, but more variable is the position of individual amino acids. The levels of amino acid in the plasma differ just a little, though. Signals of amino acids and growth factor/insulin signals are thought to converge on the mTOR pathway-also called the nutrient signalling master regulator.

Therefore, during autophagy, components of old cells are broken down into the amino acid portion (the protein building block). Does that happen to amino acids like this? The amino acid levels begin to rise in the early stages of starvation. Some amino acids derived from autophagy are believed to be provided for gluconeogenesis to the liver. These can also be broken down into glucose through the cycle of the tricarboxylic acid (TCA). The third potential fate of amino acids will be introduced into new proteins.

Two major problems – Alzheimer's Disease (AD) and cancer – will see the effects of storing old junky proteins all over the place.

Alzheimer's disease involves the accumulation of excessive protein-either amyloid-beta or Tau protein that gums the brain structure upwards. Although there is no evidence of clinical trials for this yet, it would make sense that a mechanism such as autophagy that has the ability to clean out old protein would prevent AD from developing.

What deactivates autophagy? Eating. Glucose, insulin (or glucagon decreased), and proteins all switching this self-cleaning cycle off. And it doesn't need a number. Even a tiny amount of amino acid (leucine) could stop autophagy. This cycle of autophagy is also peculiar to fasting-something that is not present in simple caloric restriction or diet.

There is, of course, a balance here. You get sick both because of too much autophagy and too little. That takes us back to life's natural cycle-fast and festive. Not smooth diet. This allows the growth of cells during eating, and cellular cleaning during fasting-balance. Life is all about balance.

HEALTH EFFECTS OF AUTOPHAGY

Evidence has associated autophagy with a variety of health effects, but this cellular process is complex, so concluding can be difficult.

A recent 2019 study, for example, surveys current autophagy and cancer studies. It finds that while autophagy can help to stop the development of cancer cells, depending on the tumour level, it can also encourage their growth.

The relation between autophagy and liver health is also of interest to the researchers. A review article in 2020 discussed ways in which autophagy would help protect the liver cells from liver damage caused by drugs and alcohol.

Other studies note that autophagy plays a role in several liver functions and may prevent many liver conditions from progressing, including:

- Wilson's disease
- Acute liver injury
- The non-alcoholic liver fatty disease
- Chronic liver disorder related to alcohol

However, most autophagy experiments occurred in test tubes or animal models. As the authors of the above research suggest, further human research is required to decide how autophagy can affect care.

By filtering out toxins and infectious agents, autophagy also tends to play an important role in the immune system.

There is evidence that autophagy by regulating inflammation could boost the outlook for cells with infectious and neurodegenerative diseases.

Another analysis article states that autophagy helps protect cells from microbes coming in.

Although there is much work on the impact of autophagy on cells, researchers are still unsure as to whether improving autophagy may be a potential therapy for different conditions.

THE AUTOPHAGY CONNECTION TO FASTING

Autophagy happens naturally within the body, but many people wonder if using specific triggers, they could induce autophagy.

Fasting is a potential autophagy-trigger. When someone fasts, they willingly go for long periods without food — hours or even a day or more.

Fasting is distinct from conventional caps on calories. When a person reduces their calories, they lower their daily food intake.

Fasting may or may not result in a limit on calories, depending on how much food a person eats during feeding times.

A 2018 review of the current literature strongly indicates that autophagy can be caused by both fasting and calorie restriction.

While some evidence of this mechanism is present in humans, the majority of these studies included non-human animals.

Restriction on fasts and calories imposes tension on the cells of the body. When a person reduces the amount of food entering their body, their cells receive fewer calories than they need for proper functioning.

When that happens, the cells have to work more effectively. Autophagy causes the cells of the body to clean out and recycle any unnecessary or damaged parts, in response to the stress caused by fasting or calorie restriction.

However, scientists are unsure as to which cells are responding in this way to fasting and calorie restrictions. For example, people who seek to trigger autophagy by fasting should be aware that this does not target fat cells.

Researchers are still debating whether fasting can provoke brain autophagy. At least one animal study indicates short-term fasting in brain cells may cause autophagy.

Can you give in to autophagy?

Restricting fasts and calories both cause autophagy by placing cells under tension. Researchers, however, assume there might be other methods of inducing autophagy.

Exercise

Exercising also puts tension on the cells of the body. When people do exercise, their cell components get weakened and inflamed. One paper's authors explain that autophagy helps our cells respond to this issue.

Which suggests people might use exercise to cause autophagy. At the same time, there is evidence that exercise in human skeletal muscles improves autophagy.

Curcumin

Researchers have also suggested that intake of curcumin triggers autophagy, at least in studies involving mice. Curcumin is a naturally occurring chemical contained in the root of the turmeric, a common spice worldwide.

For example, one animal study indicated that restored autophagy induced by curcumin might protect against diabetic cardiomyopathy, a heart muscle disease that affects people with diabetes.

Another research in mice indicated that curcumin helped combat cognitive dysfunction by inducing autophagy in some regions of the brain due to chemotherapy.

Although early results are encouraging, it is important to remember that there is a need for further work before scientists can draw any conclusions. Researchers, in particular also don't know whether increased intake of curcumin can cause autophagy in humans.

THE SIDE EFFECTS AND RISK

It is important to distinguish between the autophagy risks themselves and the risks associated with attempts by individuals to induce autophagy.

Self-autophagy isn't always optimistic. Studies have shown that excessive autophagy can kill cells in the heart, and scientists have related excessive autophagy to some heart problems.

Studies also found that inhibiting autophagy in mice could restrict tumour growth and improve cancer treatment responsiveness. This indicates that a rise in autophagy could potentially deteriorate someone's outlook with established cancer.

"Autophagy plays a complex function in cancer" and "[c] challenges and opportunities remain to recognize patients who are likely to benefit more from this approach," according to the researchers.

Many individuals are interested in using fasting and calorie restriction to cause autophagy, but little information is known about the exact impact this has on humans.

Autophagy is an important process in the body which removes damaged and unnecessary cell sections. There's evidence it can have both positive and negative effects on health.

Although studies show that dietary restriction, exercise, and intake of curcumin can affect autophagy, most studies have been performed on non-human animals.

Scientists have no full picture of the health effects of autophagy, nor of how individuals could cause it.

And someone who is seriously considering making changes to their lifestyle to cause autophagy should seek advice from a doctor in advance.

Chapter 8: HOW TO USE MINDFULNESS FOR WEIGHT LOSS

As we have already looked briefly, research supports the idea that carefulness helps individuals to maintain or achieve weight loss.

Longitudinal research has also found carefulness in helping participants reduce their Body Mass Index (BMI) significantly compared to a control group.

For this study, participants were asked to attend four two-hour carefulness workshops daily to help them understand and use awareness strategies to enhance their health and well-being. Data were collected on their BMI, physical activity, and mental wellbeing at baseline (before attending workshops), four months, and six months.

The researchers' workshops were in-depth and encouraged participants to explore their weight loss journey's emotional and physical purpose.

The guiding principles of healthy eating refer to weight loss when reaching consciousness. Also, I reviewed the overall content of the workshops used in the above study, and the following description was developed:

- Identify your values and whether weight loss supports them. Is your weight loss wish driven personally or socially motivated?
- Start understanding your food-related feelings as just that- thoughts. They need not always be believed or acted upon.
- Accept that trying to control hunger-related feelings and physical sensations won't always be successful.
- Learn how to welcome, rather than resist, internal frustration during the weight loss journey.
- Build a sense of self that enables negative thoughts and emotions around the weight loss journey to be unattached. Recognize the thoughts, but don't let them dictate how you physically respond.

- Focus on your values and attach your weight loss targets to those values.

Chocolate mentality: Guided meditation

At first glance, chocolate alertness might sound like activity of self-indulgence.

Recalling that mindfulness has, at its core, a fundamental purpose of fostering self-compassion, the idea of using chocolate in this way can become an enjoyable and valuable practice (Penman, 2011).

Mindspace has created several resources that can be used within schools to encourage the practice of mindfulness and are a great starting point for their resources for guided chocolate meditation.

I summarized their Guide below:

- Choose a small slice of candy or cookies. There can be chocolate that you're familiar with or something you've never had before—mind to approach the task with enthusiasm and transparency. Just sit down comfortably.
- Try wrapping chocolate on top of it. Can it make a sound when holding it in your hand? Which color are these? What is on the wrapper?
- Unwrap the candy, gradually. Be careful how your body starts reacting to the eating anticipation. What physical sensations do they produce? How do you emotionally react?
- Ward off the urge to eat chocolate. Instead, look at it to its fullness. You should see what colors? What does it feel like in your hand? Why it smells?
- Take a bite next, but don't just eat it yet. Close your eyes and focus on the full chocolate sensation on your tongue. Why does this look like it's melting? How does your body respond, and not just within your mouth?
- Start slowly pushing the chocolate around in your mouth. Start noticing how that tastes. How does that sense of consistency? How did this change from the time you put it on your tongue first? What thoughts do you feel?

- Swallow the chocolate once you've considered this, paying attention to the sensation as it moves down your throat. Does your tongue have a lingering taste? How do your emotions react to that?
- Put your eyes open. Take a moment to ponder how physically and emotionally, you feel.

It may sound self-indulgent, as mentioned, but taking this time to enjoy this experience can help with the ways we think about different foods. If you were always taught to think of chocolate as 'naughty,' you might have begun to indulge in eating it in secret.

This method will help to correct any flawed assumptions about how we were taught to feel about food and re-establish our enjoyment.

More Mindful Exercises to Try

Guided Meditation Mindfulness with Chocolate is a popular exercise in mindfulness; for obvious reasons! Yet you needn't use candy. Any fruits, nuts, or other small items work just as well, so changing up how you do this meditation is a good idea.

If you want to try something new, three more careful eating exercises are listed below:

1. Dinner table Mindful eating script

The following is a short script that you can work through at any meal to practice mindful eating.

- You may use or condense the full script, practice it on your own, or with friends and family who may also be interested in exploring careful eating. It can make excellent discussions at the dinner table!
- Breath in. You are now turning your focus toward your hunger or thirst for physical signals. What does it say to you? Would you feel filled up? If you feel hungry, what is it that your body wants? What are you thirsty for when you

feel thirsty? Keep all your concentration on those sensations until you hear the answers.

- Bring your attention to the food and drink on the table in front of you and imagine that for the very first time you see it. What do you immediately notice? What details await revealing? Engage all the senses and note the various colors, forms, textures, and sizes. What is it you can smell? How does your body respond to that?

- Take a moment to reflect on what the food had to go through to be on the table before you start to taste. Where was it growing? How long has it taken for this? What kind of environments were needed? Let yourself feel gratitude for the process and appreciation for everyone involved in your food journey to find their way to your table.

- Next, start savoring your food. Choose one object and explore it, adding colors, textures, and unusual smells. Note any possible emotional or physical responses. If you have any memories of this goodness? How does that make you feel? When did you taste it first?

- Turn your focus on how your body physically responds. Is your mouth watering? Does your stomach groan? How does it feel to imagine tasting the food?

- Put food inside your mouth now. Bring your consciousness into your mouth as you start chewing. Notice the textures and the flavor. Why can these later when you're already chewing? How does your body respond to that? Swallow the piece of food when you're ready, and remember the route it takes from your mouth to your stomach.

- Keep your breath stable, and repeat as you eat your meal. If you eat with others who are also taking part in the exercise, you might want to pause to share your experiences.

2. The Two-Plate Mindful Eating Approach

Mindful eating has been linked to weight loss, and if you are considering using this tool in your healthy eating journey, this next exercise might help.

The Two-Plate Mindful Eating Solution is particularly useful for those dining circumstances where, in a buffet restaurant, for example, you do not have much control over what happens on your plate. We also don't want to settle for food on our social life, and the exercise will help you find the balance for both.

Here are the effects:

- Next time you 're in a situation where you want to keep your portions under control and focus more consciously on what you're eating, pick up two plates—one to eat from and another to use as your 'serving' dish.
- Complete your serving plate with food you wish to eat.
- Take a moment's pause before you continue to serve. Bring your attention back to the breath and keep yourself grounded at the moment. Pay attention to your physical sensations when responding to the food that is before you.
- Shift some food from the serving plate to the 'eating' plate. Do not overload your plate, and listen as much as possible to your intestines. What foods appeal the most? How much would you like to eat of these?
- Start by cutting the food on your plate, pay attention while you do, concentrating on the various colors, odors, and textures. Say the mantra as you do this, 'I'm about to eat.'
- Now work your way through the plated food and take comfort, deliberate bites. Focus once again on the various sensations-physical and emotional-as you eat your food. You can also repeat the 'I am eating' mantra.
- After finishing eating this initial food plate, take a break. Bring your focus back into your body and breathe. How are you feeling? What feelings do my gut and stomach give me? Am I still thirsty, or hungry? Do I need any more food?
- If your body tells you they are still hungry, repeat the above steps. If you feel satiated, you should take away the rest of the food on the serving tray.

3.   Where Is My Food From? Reflection Training

It is a perfect exercise of mindfulness to use for children to help them (and you) become more aware and conscious of where food comes from. Practicing appreciation is a central component of mindfulness, so it makes sense to integrate that into mindful eating will help us become more aware and thankful for our meals.

Here are a few ways of learning the concept:

• Start by talking to your children about their food thoughts in a more general way. Questions for discovery could include:

- Where's your food coming from?
- How is your food growing, and what do you think it needs to help it grow?
- When did the food arrive in the supermarket?
- Why do you think those things are important to think about?

• Use some of its answers to improve your next activities. Before this, you may want to do some work yourself, or you may want to use it as a learning tool that you share. May include: Exploration events

- A visit to the local farmers ' market to ask farmers where they live and produce sellers, how they grow their favorite foods, and how long it takes.
- A visit to a fruit orchard to pick up your fruit and learn how the fruit grows, what seasons it's best to eat in, and ask the staff questions.
- Plan to make more scratched meals, such as sauces, cakes, and biscuits, to explore the 'making' aspect of various foods.
- Check where your favorite food is in the fruit and vegetable aisle or on the back of the packets at your local supermarket-is is it locally grown or far away?
- Start a patch of vegetables in the garden or indoor herb garden to explore the growing things yourself.
- Next time you 're having a meal, encourage ongoing reflection, and continue the conversation. When you have selected or grown fruit and vegetables, practice a moment of appreciation or celebration.

Chapter 9: THE TOP 10 REASONS TO USE HYPNOTHERAPY WEIGHT LOSS

The top 10 reasons to use hypnotherapy for weight loss

What is Hypnotherapy for Weight Loss?

Hypnotherapy to weight loss is used much more common than most people will know. Hypnosis is not something people do on Television shows that put them to sleep immediately, but a medical technique that has a much broader scope of positive results.

Hypnotherapy for weight loss is used in a range of weight-related treatments such as binge eating and bulimia but also helps to treat trigger symptoms such as anxiety.

Here are ten top reasons for using hypnotherapy for weight loss as a choice or in favor of a diet regulated with calories.

Hypnosis fundamentally changes your way of thinking regarding food

Hypnosis therapy works by subconsciously placing educational suggestions in the recipients with the sole purpose of changing the habits of that person. Your therapist will change the way that you focus on food, portion size, and trigger points when using this for weight loss.

It doesn't make you want to eat extra food or treat

The mind conditioning hypnotherapy for weight loss provides you with the transition from snacking or treating yourself to the usual cakes, sweets, or chocolates that ruin your balanced diet.

Hypnotherapy operates by re-training the brain to imagine the desired future weight and body form for weight loss. It then serves as a trigger and motivator built-in

Eating the right food is automatic

The power of hypnotherapy will allow you to work upfront in selecting the right foods, not relying on fad diets, binge eating, or relying on sweet foods or taking away foods.

You are encouraged to feel good about eating less

Hypnotherapy should encourage you to choose the right portion size for your meals without getting hungry again after the thought. Incorrect portion sizes are one of the main weight gain contributors.

Less food makes you feel more satisfied

You should see a decrease in your weight by reducing your portion size and efficiently taking in calories. Eating smaller drinks would not only please you but also make you feel better about yourself.

It promotes a general change of attitude which includes motivation for regular physical exercise

Many of my customers first come to the food for a change of attitude. Once they find that they have achieved the mental outlook that can be achieved by a positive approach to food, a natural progression to sports or gym soon follows, and their confidence about their weight loss is increasing.

It replaces the old thought loop with a new attitude of trust and optimistic "can do."

Many individuals who undergo hypnotherapy do so unsurely of what the results would be. With hypnotherapy, there are no assurances as just as for a diet program; there are no assurances. Results may differ by person.

However, we see patients use weight loss hypnotherapy regularly very effectively, and they break their old thought loop and build a mindset of "can do" without being pushed into it.

This makes weight loss possible by reverting the subconscious mind

Weight loss hypnotherapy is designed to get your subconscious mind to have already decided to eat well, take the right portion size, take the right foods, and even encourage a positive feeling when doing all that.

Reconnecting the subconscious mind is a strong resource for weight loss and many other hypnotherapy-treated behaviors.

Less becomes more the new motto of mind

Hypnotherapy for weight-loss allows you to accept that less is more. By this, we mean when you first pick the right mental portion size but see the plate as usually much smaller than you're used to, it won't feel odd or uncomfortable or build a mentality of thinking "that's not enough."

The old finish your plate mentality is replaced by I don't have to finish my plate; your long-term appetite is fundamentally reduced

Overeating, as well as portion size, is another form of self-abuse when it comes to managing our weight. Weight loss hypnotherapy allows the patient to move away from a mentality of "I see, I eat," to a more controlled way of eating that responds to the body telling you its fullness.

Who is hypnotherapy for weight loss meant for?

Hypnotherapy for Weight Loss is for everyone. Results are not standardized and depend on the person involved. Will strength, motivation, approach, and need will play a part in the result, but still, significant consideration should be given to hypnosis.

Want to lose some weight?

Thousands of people just feel like you are doing right now. Christmas was and was gone, the festivities brought a few extra pounds, and the drinking sessions from there seemed to have continued.

Yet deep down, you know that you're not very pleased with what's happening, and you want to change that.

Up to now, diets may not have worked for you, but you're willing to try something that can give you the optimistic edge you need to regulate the cravings around food.

Understand why diets alone do not hold weight loss effective

Hypnotherapy protects your diet by:

- Subconscious suggestion planting
- Letting go of the need to cheat
- Discover why diet doesn't change your habits
- Hypnosis has proven to help weight loss.

Many people need to understand that a bad or unhealthy diet is usually the result of years of constant food consumption training.

Late work, lack of access to safe, acceptable alternatives, lifestyle, and lack of awareness of what's good and what doesn't contribute.

Weight loss

Losing weight can be a difficult process-not facilitated by the world's conflicting, and often dangerous, advice out there. We are continually bombarded with television programs, ads, and social media feeds full of food images. The presence of these can make the desire very powerful to turn away from safe or intuitive eating.

Then there are pills for weight loss and other programs for reducing commercial weight that focus on restricting what you eat, rather than considering how you eat or what you think about the food you put in your body. It is no surprise that certain negative mindsets have developed around what we put in our bodies.

Weight loss hypnosis can be a successful way of questioning these mentalities and moments of temptation, allowing you to lead a healthy life.

Weight loss hypnotherapy aims to make you feel good about your body, shift unhealthy eating thoughts, and help you lose weight responsibly, without impacting your emotional well-being. Through using effective persuasion methods to reach the unconscious mind, a hypnotherapist may help you build a positive relationship with food and exercise, which is essential to safe weight loss and long-term weight control.

Will I lose weight?

Many people insist they need to lose weight, whether they are overweight or not. But the fact is, very few people are content with their body shape and appearance regardless of whether they need to lose weight.

Trust to the body

While people need to lose weight if they are overweight for health reasons, it is not healthy to feel ashamed of the need or the urge to lose weight. Because the shape and size of the body are so tied to the western idea of beauty, people are constantly looking for 'quick fixes' to cut angles.

Pills for weight loss, fad diets, and grueling fitness routines are just a couple of the ways people seek to lose weight. What must you ask yourself is-am I happy to do this? Will I afford to do that for the rest of my life?

Here's where weight loss hypnotherapy can help. You need to change your mind first, to change your body. You must ask yourself, why am I dissatisfied with my body, and why am I not able to lose weight?

To learn more about how low self-confidence can boost hypnotherapy, please visit our factsheet.

How does Weight Loss Hypnosis work?

Weight loss hypnotherapy is becoming more common, and people around the world are finding it beneficial to maintain a healthy weight in the long term.

With time and a series of weight loss hypnotherapy sessions-you'll learn how to substitute your hypnotherapist 's recommended unhealthy habits and to eat behaviors with the better ones.

What happens with weight loss during the hypnosis?

Your hypnotherapist will guide you into a deeply relaxed state.

When your body and mind are completely relaxed, the hypnotherapist should be able to reach the unconscious mind (the part of us that operates all the time but we are not consciously aware of, that is, instincts and mechanisms of survival).

Soothing, carefully worded scripts can be used to analyze the motives for overeating a client and, through visualizations, propose new ways of thought. Without any input from your hypnotherapist, you have the power to ignore any suggestions you do not feel comfortable with. For some of the techniques and visualizations that they may use, see below.

Hypnotherapy to techniques for weight loss

While each case is different because everyone has their reasons to want to lose weight, there are some suggestions you may encounter:

- Imagine the body you like, or the fitness/health standard that you want to achieve.
- Imagine how the new look and health will make you feel.
- Imagine effortlessly achieving that goal yourself.
- See how far you'll have gotten away from today.
- Imagine how energized and confident you are about to feel.
- Realizing that the more you practice, the more you want to exercise, the easier it becomes to do so.

These strategies are designed to motivate you to get control of your decisions. However, if you're worried that your relationship with certain types of food becomes unhealthy, food addiction hypnotherapy might help you break these negative thinking patterns.

You can learn to love the taste of healthy food by weight loss hypnosis, and avoid eating sugar, fatty foods. Also, you should learn to love your body and not see it as a source of concern. Hypnosis for weight loss can help you adopt a healthier, happier, lifestyle and mindset by tackling those deep feelings that form the foundations of your eating habits.

Its potential points of weight loss

Lots of people try and for a variety of reasons don't lose weight. Such causes are mostly latent, otherwise known as 'secondary benefits,' which makes it impossible for us to solve these.

If anyone works on weight loss, the illusion that has held the weight in place for so long is worth looking at. We always hold convictions on two levels; at the conscious level, we think positive thoughts about ourselves, our worth, and what we as human beings deserve, but unconsciously, our actions give away our emotional convictions about ourselves.

The fact is, sometimes we can gain comfort by not making changes-we feel comfortable to remain just as we are. So, we may actively want to lose weight, but we are stopped by something in the subconscious from making it a reality. Weight loss hypnotherapy aims to expose these reasons, allowing clients to finally break through barriers that may have prevented them from losing weight for many years.

Below we'll take a look at some of the reasons you may find it difficult to lose weight successfully.

You feel relaxed eating

When we are babies, we learn how to equate feeding with our

mothers' comfort. Some experts claim that this connection never really leaves us, and we can return to those early days of total dependency when life becomes stressful. It is here that emotional eating can become a problem.

If, after a long day, you've ever found yourself hitting a candy bar or ordering a takeaway when you're feeling lonely and sad, you may be a relaxed eater. You'll find it difficult to lose weight as a comfort eater because you've let food become your coping mechanism, and, without it, you may not know how to cope with your emotions.

Hypnotherapy will help you cope with this, helping you learn how to handle negative feelings in a way that does not contribute to eating comfort.

The biggest change is that I got a lot less bothered with eating. I still love eating because when my body is hungry, I've learned to feed and not only because my subconscious needs something to soothe my emotions.

You eat mindlessly

You have to be honest about how much you eat and exercise to lose weight. Even if you keep a food diary or use a food-tracking app, the odd snack here and there can be easily forgotten. Maybe you are picking ingredients while you're making dinner? Do you grab something to work on your walk, or tuck your afternoon tea into a biscuit?

It is often these foods 'on the go' that catch us out, but they add up. Even if you faithfully stick to the salad for dinner, you won't do any favors to forget all the things that you eat in between. This kind of reckless eating is something that weight loss hypnotherapy will help you get through.

If you are struggling with mindful eating, gastric band hypnotherapy may help. The idea is to make you feel fuller for longer, which can help in preventing constant grazing all day long.

You ban foodstuffs

You're told not to open up like a mysterious box, eliminating certain foods from your diet can make them all the more appealing. If you find yourself restricting the food you eat, when your willpower takes a dip, you are more likely to want to get binge.

Learning mindful eating is the secret to consistent and safe weight loss. When you can eat attentively and savor every bite, then you will be able to enjoy your favorite food in moderation and prevent weight loss.

Significantly, encouraging clients to eat deliberately is a vital aspect of hypnosis for weight loss-placing emotional factors aside and cultivating a positive relationship with food that encourages a balanced, long-term weight.

You don't get out enough

If it comes to weight loss, exercise is just as critical as diet. The mental blocks can often stop us from exercising, including:

- Feeling powerless
- Too self-conscious to go out in public
- Convincing yourself (every day) that you'll 'go tomorrow.

Hypnotherapy for weight loss will help you break down the mental barriers that stop you from making the most of your body. More often than not, rotating your body and beating your heart will help you feel better overall about yourself, leading to longer-term healthy habits and satisfaction.

Can hypnosis appeal to me for weight loss?

One of the most commonly asked questions in seminars about hypnotherapy is-does hypnotherapy function for me for weight loss? It's hard to know the answer to that until you try it out yourself. Although it definitely won't work the same way for everyone, thinking about creating healthy habits and getting rid of poor habits will help to build a new level of consciousness about diet and exercise.

It is important to remember that hypnotherapy is a complementary therapy and should, therefore, be used in conjunction with a healthy eating plan and exercise regime. If you want advice on better eating and exercising, it might be useful to talk to your doctor or a nutrition professional. Often it's a combined effort of all these things which leads to success.

Chapter 10: ERRORS IN WEIGHT LOSS YOU NEED TO STOP MAKING

Here are nine weight loss mistakes to avoid making today:

1. Asking yourself that you are going to resume Monday again.

This is an extremely common dietary mistake that millions of people make every week, and I was there too. However, it would just end up holding you off your weight loss target forever, leaving you trapped on the "someday-Monday-itis" daily hamster wheel.

Why would it stop you from weight loss? For all the overeating and unhealthy living you do before Monday through the week is just your lifestyle. Unfortunately, it's just not enough two days of healthy eating per week to get you to your goal weight and keep you there.

2. Wait till New Year's Day.

This is another super common mistake made every holiday season by millions upon millions of overweight overeaters. Yeah, I know too how easy it is between Thanksgiving and New Year's Day to pack on 20 pounds! In reality, I was just thinking about this with one of my weight loss coaching clients (she's the one who said earning 20 pounds would be easy and quick before January 1st!).

It is such a big mistake to make — to try to make a New Year's weight loss goal.

Not only would you be heavier on January 1st, but you'll also add to the momentum of the overeating and overindulgence 500 mph freight train that you've been riding through.

How on 1st January do you stop a speeding train on its tracks? Isn't it more common for a freight train just to continue? And then? After all, Valentine's Day is right around the corner, and then Easter is coming up that birthday, wedding, holiday ... So then, before you know it, it's a year later, so you promise yourself that you're going to continue on New Year's Day 2018 again.

What if you now stop doing this for yourself? What if you just go ahead with your action plan on weight loss? Only make sure you have the right program in place to feed your mind every day before your body. It is the puzzle's most critical piece (more on that below).

3. Eat when you don't feel hungry.

Your body has no choice but to store that extra food as fat when you put food in your mouth when your stomach is not empty.

Why? For what? Okay, imagine driving your car to the gas station at a full tank. How can you get gas inside your car?

On this Earth, your car (that's your body) doesn't need fuel because it's already loaded. Food is combustible. Getting "good times" with, or date is not something. So when you feed only when you're physically thirsty, your body can't resist shedding the extra fat!

4. Trying to make it fine.

Possibly you have heard the saying, "Development not perfection," right? Well, when it comes to weight loss and keeping it off, it is real. Although you need to move towards your perfect body, most of the time, one slip up a month or so is not an excuse to throw in the towel.

Just stand up and get back on track — this is what those with a mindset about weight loss do! They just don't make it a big deal about it, and so from one slip up, it doesn't cost them weight gain.

5. Expect to lose 20 pounds in 20 days (or some other kind of mad instant weight loss gratification thing).

If you're overweight 500 pounds, you just won't lose 20 pounds in

20 days. I know you see these crazy claims about diet pills and cleanses and so on, but even if you could lose weight so easily, I guarantee you wouldn't lose fat.

That's why it comes back right in the blink of an eye as soon as you quit doing a cleanse trick or another "quick fat loss."

6. Believing in the fairy tales about weight loss.

I 'm sorry to break it down for you, but there's no magic pill, powder, cleanse or shake that will help you shed fat and keep it away forever while you're still living the same lifestyle you 're living today.

Yep! Yea! That is what individuals are looking for. Trying to lose weight every day while eating pizza and ice cream, making no changes to their diet and exercise routines while popping up a magic weight loss pill to cure it all.

(Ack! I know how easy it is when you're desperate to lose weight to believe that stuff! Sadly that stuff just doesn't work.)

Here's the truth: A safe, consistent lifestyle is the only permanent weight loss "trick" that works. This is it! Practice a safe day in and day out lifestyle, and you'll make it.

But if you want to be able to do it, do it regularly, and for it to be fun and simple, then you need the biggest piece of the equation for good weight loss: an attitude about weight loss.

7. Leaving 'Universal Rules' off the path of weight loss.

If you believe in this Universe's rules or not, it doesn't change the fact that they are what they are. You will continue fighting an uphill battle if you leave Universal Laws out of your weight loss journey.

One of the Universal Laws under which we all live, which perfectly illustrates what I mean, is: "You can not enjoy the outcome of a journey you despise."

Here's a good example: if you hate healthy eating and exercise, you won't be satisfied until you lose weight even though you can get yourself to do it! Now you have to be comfortable, right where you are, as you move with ease into your perfect body.

If you are mentality about weight loss, it's easy to lose weight. It could not be any other way. So your mindset is so powerful. This either keeps working to make your body overweight (that's what an overweight mentality is supposed to do) or if you have an attitude about weight loss, it will work to get the body fit and lean with struggle-free, balanced behaviors. Simple and intimate!

Remember that if you feel disappointed after reading this because you've never had a simple, enjoyable weight loss, it's only because you don't have the right attitude. The positive thing is that it will turn your attitude into a perspective on weight loss. So everything is fine!

8. Telling yourself, "I 'm going to go there alone."

When you struggle with emotional eating, binge eating, food addiction, low self-esteem, self-doubts, night-time eating, and the inability to stop stuffing yourself, but you keep saying to yourself, "I 'm going to go it alone. I'm just going to make myself do it!"—how exactly does that work for you?

This is a costly mistake to make when you could get help from a proven, professional weight loss coach who already has the proven step-by-step system to end your food and weight struggles.

The quickest and easiest way to achieve the weight loss results that you want is to train with the right coach. Based on my observations since I started coaching in 2009, I've never had a weight loss coaching client telling me they've been able to get the results they have been working with me alone. Since they can't. Why? For what? Because we can't see any of our blind spots. And, the right permanent weight loss coach can see yours and help you crack them out!

Especially if she is an intuitive trainer too.

9. Ignoring permanent weight loss as the largest honking piece of a solution.

An attitude about weight loss is the largest honking component of the solution to sustainable weight loss. It's so big it's difficult to lose weight without it.

Mindset is 92.8 percent of the problem when eating can't stop. When you want to lose weight and hold it off, that's 92.8 percent of the answer too.

Your subconscious is in control of your body. Ever.

Your behaviors will be fat when your mindset is fat, and your body will match. See how it works?

If you're stopping making these nine weight loss errors and moving forward now, just think about where you could be in six months.

Healthy feeding: how healthy feeding will boost overall health

What is Sensitive Eating?

There is a propensity to believe that learning will take place in a quiet environment. Still, the essence of the activity also translates with wonderful benefits into more active areas of daily life.

One field that you might not have considered applying the procedure could be your eating habits.

It is common for our timetables to be overwhelming in our busy and tech-focused lives. Forgetting to eat lunch is not uncommon. Or if we remember to feed, if we give our body what it wants, we choke our meal down, without even thought.

How often did you eat a meal afterward, only to feel hungry? Rarely will we allow the opportunity to our brains and bodies to process the fact that food has arrived or has taken the time to appreciate mealtime presence.

According to the Mindful Eating Center, mindful eating combines meditation and mindfulness practice to help you understand what you eat when you eat, why you eat and enjoy food when you eat it.

Through practicing healthy eating, you will become more conscious of your food patterns-good, and poor-and make the required adjustments to enhance your sense of well-being that can be accomplished by food. It's a way to listen to the hallmarks of your body to recognize when you're hungry, thirsty, satiated, and the nutrients it craves.

Initially, a team of 19 counseling and therapy practitioners at the Center for Mindful Eating created the concepts of mindful eating. They 're a great base from which to develop your knowledge in this area. The Centre 's services are vast, but some general aspects of cautious eating include:

- Engage all the senses while selecting which foods to consume and pay attention to how it looks, feels, smells, and tastes.
- I have time for deliberately choosing, planning, and cooking meals.
- Beware of how the body physically reacts to various foods.
- Increase understanding of the signs that direct and remind you when to eat and when to avoid eating.

Anyone who uses mindfulness practice when eating:

- Accepts that there is no wrong or right way of eating, but there are different levels of awareness regarding the eating experience.

- Recognizes that eating experiences are unique to everyone.
- Sensitize how their eating habits can support their overall health and well-being.
- Understands the profound interrelationship that exists between all living beings, cultural dynamics, and how food choices affect these connections.

Mindful eating reaches beyond the adult and accepts the awareness of how and what you eat has a wider influence on the environment (Cheung, 2016).

THE BENEFITS OF CONSCIENTIOUS EATING

One of the most important advantages of cautious eating is how it can help you make healthy food decisions that have many roll-on effects. Even generic practices of mindfulness can significantly impact healthy eating habits (Jordan et al., 2014).

1. Energy loss

One of the benefits of mindful eating reported more widely is weight loss. Mindful eating was related to weight control and active weight loss in people who were labeled as obese (Dalen et al ., 2010) and also had success for women who report regularly eating in restaurant settings where the practice of mindfulness might be more difficult (Timmerman & Brown, 2012).

Another research showed that people who consume more deliberately report consuming smaller serving sizes of high-calorie foods, helping their weight loss journeys (Beshara, Hutchinson, & Wilson, 2013).

Unlike typical dietary methods that can create feelings of deprivation, careful eating encourages you to connect deeply with the physical need for food and the negative impact of overeating the wrong foods on the mind and body.

2. Wellbeing and other psychological advantages

Eating carefully also helps to encourage psychological health. Different foods may have a direct effect on our emotional states (Kidwell & Hasford, 2014), so you exercise better control over your mental well-being while approaching eating with mindfulness.

Some advantages of cautious eating may include:

- It recognizes patterns of emotional and reactive eating, which lead to poor emotional health.
- Body, heart, mind, and soul nutrition;
- Increased understanding of the interaction with food and the wider climate.
- Better control and confidence to make healthy, deliberate decisions.

HOW TO PRACTICE FOOD MINDFULNESS

Practicing food consciousness can take some effort, but making incremental changes will make a significant difference over time.

It's about taking stock of daily activities that we normally brush by, taking the time to act deliberately, and paying attention to our surroundings and physical presence within them, as with any practice of mindfulness.

I have read thoroughly through some of the studies and countless blog posts to compile a list of ten tips below to help you get started with a careful eating practice:

1. Start with your shopping list-write a comprehensive shopping list before you start shopping. Remember the health benefits of everything you put on that list; it's sustainability and nutritious value in your kitchen pantry. Be sure that when you're hungry, you don't shop (which can lead to transactions of impulses) and stick to

your plan.

2. Prepare for success-think ahead of the week and plan accordingly. When we have a busy schedule and have not prepared for our meals, it can be easy to turn to fast foods, foods that we know don't offer us a lot of nutrition or no food at all.

3. Document hunger and act on it – This one will take some practice. How much do you listen to the clues your body gives you what it wants in the week? It's a common mistake that when our body tries to tell us it's thirsty, we often think we are hungry (Mattes, 2010). Spend some time understanding the signs your body is giving you better, and acting appropriately on them.

4. Do not wait until you are hungry to eat. If you skip meals and wait to give your body what it needs, you will come to the hungry table, which usually leads to eating and overeating impulses as you try to fill the void of hunger instead of eating meaningfully. This returns to tip number two – always get ready for busy days and make time to eat.

5. Consider your portion size – Starting with a smaller portion size will help you become more aware of the food that's actually on your plate and increase your concentration on what you're consuming and how it satisfies your hunger needs.

6. Create a mealtime accompanying ritual – Research has found that even blowing the candles out on a birthday cake has shown an improvement in how it tastes (Vohs et al . , 2013). If it's saying grace, offering thanks, or simply arranging your cutlery and napkin in a specific way, a little routine before you start eating will make a huge difference in how you enjoy your meal.

7. Eat engaged with all your senses – turn off the television, put away your phone, save the book for later – when you're sitting down at a meal, give it your total undivided attention. Engage every

meal with all your senses-how does it smell? Which textures are different? What are the colors in that? How does the food feel in your stomach, on your tongue? Taste the first bite, and enjoy every moment.

8. Take a break between bites – Taking a break between bites is another way to bring your attention to your meal. Put down your utensils and take a break as you complete your mouthful. Before continuing with your meal, reflect on the food left on your plate. This allows you to slow down mentally and gives you the chance to check in with your body and see how your fullness levels are doing.

9. Chew slowly and pay attention – It's too easy to inhale your food on a busy working day, and move on to the next thing. Beware of taking this slowly – and that includes the physical movement of eating itself. Make a deliberate effort to chew more slowly than you would normally. How much you taste and how much faster you feel full can surprise you.

10. Take the time to reflect – mindfulness doesn't end when your meal is finished. Take a moment to remember how you feel about food now. Listen to your body and take note of the different sensations and emotional reactions that eating has brought.

Chapter 11: STOPPING FOOD ADDICTION

Food is something that we all need to survive, nourishing us, fueling us, and contributing to our health and wellness. In an ideal world, we would all eat a varied, balanced diet that both physically and emotionally fulfills us. However, food is sad, a complicated subject.

Some of us can establish unhealthy relationships with food, use it in unhelpful ways, and create a behavioral addiction in some cases. Highly palatable foods (i.e., those high in fat, sugar, or salt) cause a chemical reaction within the brain, causing a sense of gratification and satisfaction.

This reaction can get addictive for anyone with an unhealthy food relationship. Though the eating disorder is not known to be 'food addiction,' having this kind of relationship with food can lead to physical and psychological difficulties. Here we will go deeper into the concept of food addiction and how hypnotherapy can help you develop a safer, happier relationship with food.

What is Addiction to Food?

In the diet industry, there's a lot of controversy over whether or not food addiction is actual. Brain imaging and other studies of people with 'food addictions' have shown similar outcomes to those with alcohol addictions. Unlike drug addiction, however, food addiction is not a chemical dependency; it's a behavioral dependency.

People are therefore not addicted to food per se, but rather to the act of eating and the feeling they get after feeding. This appears to be improved by highly palatable foods, as they release feel-good chemicals, such as dopamine, into the brain.

People who develop this behavioral problem can be obsessed with food and eating thoughts. They can experience shameful feelings after eating too. Eating those foods also comes with a side of guilt due to our diet culture driven society and unrealistic beauty standards, making it very difficult for people to cultivate balanced and rational attitudes towards food.

What causes addiction to food?

Like in other addictions, there is never a single cause but rather a combination of causes. It may be biological, psychological, or social influences. Biological causes include hormonal imbalances, a variation in the development of the brain, side effects of other drugs, or even a family member dealing with addictions.

Psychological factors can include witnessing trauma or violence, having trouble coping with negative feelings, having low self-esteem, or dealing with sadness or loss. When we are suffering mentally, food is also used as a soothing mechanism or coping device. If this is at the heart of your addiction, if you want to change your relationship with food, it's important to fix it.

Certain aspects of mental wellbeing can also affect poor eating behaviors. These problems include eating disorders, anxiety, and depression. If you're worried about a mental health condition, be sure to talk to your doctor or counselor, sometimes treating this can help improve your relationship with food.

Social factors that can contribute to food addiction can include family issues, peer or societal pressure, feeling isolated and stressful events in life. Not having a support system in place will make the eating problems difficult to overcome. Try reaching out and talking about how you feel, either in a support group or with friends and family.

Results of food addiction

If food addiction is left untreated, it can affect your physical and mental health considerably. Continuing to eat large amounts of foods high in sugar and salt can lead to physical complications such as heart disease, digestive problems, sleep disturbances, headaches, increased risk of stroke, and general lethargy.

Psychologically, this kind of food relationship can affect your self-esteem, which leads to conditions like depression and anxiety. You can tend to develop disordered eating and even battle suicidal thoughts.

Signs of an unhealthy food relationship

Recognizing you have an eating disorder is the first step in having help. If you think you may have an unhealthy relationship with food, here are some questions to ask.

You do:

- When it comes to other foods, you find that you consume more than planned?
- Try to eat some food even though you're not hungry?
- Feed when you are feeling unwell?
- Worry about cutting back on other foods or not consuming them?
- Do you panic when those foods are not available, or do you go out of your way to procure them?
- Finding eating gets in the way of other activities, like family time or hobbies?
- Stop social conditions where there is food for fear of overeating?
- Are you finding it hard to function because of food / eating at work/school?
- Are you feeling low, nervous, or guilty after having eaten?
- Need to eat more and more to reduce negative emotions or to boost pleasure?

When it has become a major enough concern impacting your daily life, it's always best to see medical help. Keep on reading to find out how hypnotherapy will help you.

Hypnotherapy for food abuse

The essence of food addiction and the many complex factors leading to it means that motivation alone is sometimes not enough. It is also important to understand what could affect your actions and to identify dysfunctional coping mechanisms before research can be done to improve your behavior.

Hypnotherapy is effective in improving behaviors. Your hypnotherapist will help you to reach a deeply relaxed state in which your subconscious is more likely to be suggestive.

Your hypnotherapist can work with you to discover your addiction's underlying cause before offering your subconscious suggestions to help you change habits and behaviors.

Hypnotherapy is a perfect resource for assisting you with this process because our subconscious mind is much more open to new ideas when we are thoroughly comfortable. And a trained hypnotherapist will be able to direct you through the process with a little bit of effort on your side, sometimes resulting in a much smoother improvement than willpower alone.

Hypnotherapy's calming nature will also help you become more self-aware and conscious of the food. Learning to identify hunger signals is crucial and something many of us is struggling with when you're loaded.

Your hypnotherapist should not recommend that you go on a diet or offer nutritional advice (unless they are nutritionally trained); instead, they should work with you in mindset, get to the root of the problem and help you make lasting changes.

How do I get a hypnotherapist?

If you're ready to make a change, finding a hypnotherapist that resonates with you will be the first step on your journey. We have an evidence policy in place on Hypnotherapy Directory to ensure that all the practitioners listed on our platform have received evidence of training and insurance or are members of a professional body. We also encourage our members to provide plenty of information to fill out their profiles. This allows you to learn more about how they work and whether they are the person to help.

Binge Eating hypnosis: Overcoming Food Addictions with Hypnotherapy

What is Binge Eating Hypnosis? And does it work for overeating and unhealthy eating?

Do you ever feel as though your life is about food? Food is a significant part of our everyday lives, from holidays and birthday parties to dinner time with relatives.

And we've always been conditioned to have an unhealthy food relationship. We've started to eat food, and a lot of us are eating sugar. Some, for example, use food in times of stress for warmth-they are emotional eaters. Some continually struggle to overindulge cravings. And when they get bored some change to food.

The explanation is simple: We have conditioned our subconscious to use food as a comfort blanket.

That's Okay. Our subconscious – the large information repository that controls 85-95 percent of our thoughts – wants us to feel safe. The response to fight or flight is a natural subconscious mechanism of defense; it keeps us safe when we are in danger.

Those times when we give in to the sugar temptations, the subconscious is in defense mode when we are safe. That is why we are tempted to look for snacks or overeat immediately. Our subconscious has learned that "health" is equated with sugar snacks, or the feeling overfull.

To put it another way, overcoming food addiction requires more than willpower. Yeah, you heard that right, you don't need any willpower to conquer the addiction to food. You just have to retrain your subconscious mind to support those automatic cravings and release them.

That's why hypnosis can be so effective with food addiction.

Hypnosis helps one to reach into the subconscious. And when we talk to the subconscious directly, we can begin to release bad habits and retrain our subconscious to be a supporter. Indeed it is much simpler than it looks.

You may ask, "How does hypnosis work for food dependence? "This is how you should think of it: hypnosis opens a clear communication line with the subconscious. We can speak to it directly and use it to feed positive affirmations and new information. We can reprogram our consciousness, thanks to the hypnosis.

A CLOSER LOOK

Food addiction has many clinical names, and people may have a whole host of unhealthy food relationships.

For example, binge eating disorder happens when people plan on regularly consuming an excessive amount of food. A binge eater appears to eat tens of thousands of calories in a short time, often mindlessly, and such binges have significant health implications. The urge to binge is often irrational-hypnosis helps us to manage and control these urges.

In contrast, compulsive overeating is similar. Compulsive overeaters are also overcome by cravings-most often for sugar, dairy, or carbohydrates. And according to the National Center for Eating Disorders, they experience a lack of control over their cravings. Hypnosis helps us to understand cravings, and reprogram the subconscious to be more helpful in helping to conquer overeat urges.

Some people finally call themselves sugar addicts, or carb addicts.

Cravings are for a particular product, and cravings for such unhealthy choices do not seem to blow. For example, the hypnosis of sugar addiction can help us reframe how the subconscious sees sugar, and in turn, will help us alleviate our cravings.

Many food addicts experience common symptoms, regardless of the type of addictions:

- Eating quick
- Keep feeding even though you are full
- Eats sometimes though you don't feel hungry
- Eating Secretly
- Feeling shame or regret for overconsumption
- And feeling obliged to eat, or "guided,"

And what is the cause of the unhealthy food relationship? The root causes of our food addictions lie predominantly inside the subconscious mind. For example, we have been conditioned to add positive associations to certain types of food or overeating or binging, and those associations are deeply rooted in the subconscious.

How Our feelings reinforce food addictions

Overeating, binging, or extreme cravings aren't the issue – the problem is the negative habits of thought that cause us to make unhealthy eating decisions.

Such connections are, sadly, profoundly rooted. We've spent our lives leading ourselves to unhealthy food.

Parties, marriages, baking cookies with grandma – we've discovered that our mates are sugary treats and unhealthy foods. Some of us use them to reward ourselves, relieve boredom or anxiety, even when we feel anxious, some of us eat.

And very often, our cravings are involuntarily activated. We feel pain, and we feel BAM! We reach into the cabinet and eat without knowing just why.

We often don't even consider our subconscious minds-that area where research suggests that 85-95% of brain activity lies. And this is the region of the brain where addiction to food resides.

Our subconscious thoughts are automatic and have been reinforced over a lifetime of experience. For example, we may have found comfort in food after a traumatic childhood event, learning that food has helped to numb the feelings of pain or shame. As you can see, we 're turning to comfort food!

The cravings may also be linked to positive activities. Imagine this: Someone might associate sweets with grandma baking. In effect, their subconscious associate's sweets with love and health. That's why in emotional situations, or when we're stressed, so many of us turn to food – we want comfort!

The good news: It can retrain the subconscious. Hypnosis naturally and successfully helps one preserve the subconscious. And many conditions which are caused by unhealthy patterns of thinking, such as anxiety and stress, have been shown to help.

Hypnosis will make us feel hyper-conscious of our cravings. We learn to acknowledge that. They happen so often automatically and without thinking, but when we learn to recognize them, we gain power over our cravings.

We may also use hypnosis to reach the subconscious and provide new, more useful insight into this amazing repository of knowledge. Just think of it as pulling weeds to plant new, healthy seeds. We could reframe how we think about fast food, for example, and motivate the subconscious to search for and seek healthier alternatives.

Food Addiction Hypnotherapy: How Can It Help

By now, you have an understanding of how hypnosis helps: it empowers us to be mindful of our cravings and allows the mind to focus on food. But just how does that work?

Here's a look at some of the finer food addiction hypnosis points, and some of the many ways that this can empower us to lead healthier lives.

Mindful eating: Food addictions almost all share a similar symptom: We often over-eat without thinking. This is becoming a habit and something we don't even think about. We may teach the mind to be more conscious of our cravings, how full we feel, and the actual act of eating with hypnosis for mindful feeding. Mindful eating hypnosis helps us to understand hunger cravings and physical sensations and to be mindful of food. We are gaining strength over food and our cravings.

Breaking Habitual Thoughts: Usual thought is all too frequently reactionary and pessimistic. Quite sometimes, these thoughts cause our cravings or overeating. You may encounter a stressful situation at work, and instead of taking a breath and saying it's all going to be Fine, you start feeling you 're underqualified, or the stress turns to anxiety. We can not release our food addictions without eliminating those spiraling thinking patterns. Hypnosis helps us to regain control of our emotions, and turn our subconscious into a strong ally.

Repairing Underlying Conditions: Any number of conditions can perpetuate food addiction: Depression, anxiety, lack of self-love, to name a few. Hypnosis will help us to control certain problems and move beyond them.

Restoring Trust: Lack of self-confidence or love will stop us from taking action. If we don't trust ourselves, or if we don't value ourselves, then we can allow our bad habits to continue. Hypnotherapy is a strong tool for gaining confidence and learning to love ourselves more. It is critical of food addictions. We are much more likely to experience cravings when we love and believe in ourselves and work towards making healthy lifestyle choices.

SELF-HYPNOSIS TO RELEASE BAD EATING HABITS

When it comes to hypnotherapy, people have some options: one-on-one sessions with a hypnotherapist, listening to recordings of hypnosis, and self-hypnosis. Self-hypnosis is one of the most convenient because you can use it at home or in the office.

Food addictions are also highly recommended. To learn how to use Grace's self-hypnosis, check out this video. As you can see, that is a simple operation. Here are a few things you may want to bear in mind:

Note Your Well-being: How is it that you feel? Assessing how you feel is helpful, so at the end of the session, you can reassess it.

Controlled Breathing and Visualization: Deep breathing shows that relaxation is time for the body and mind. Visualization is also another form of relaxation initiation.

A Guided Countdown: You can countdown from 10 to pick. This helps the mind enter a hypnosis-state.

Strong affirmations: You should talk directly to the subconscious when you're comfortable. Offer affirmations to it, constructive ideas for reconditioning the mind. With food addiction, for instance, you might repeat something like: "I 'm free from overeating. I listen to know my body when to eat. I prefer to eat full portions of nutritious foods. I'm avoiding sugary foods. Every single day, I feel healthier.

Visualizing the Change: Visualize the way you will be following the healthier path after you have given your subconscious positive suggestions. See yourself living on a balanced food partnership. This strengthens the idea and allows it to take hold and to sustain it.

Hypnotherapy and aversion therapy: reframing the mind

Sweet, salty, or fatty foods bring with them several side effects. Overindulgence is linked to obesity, diabetes, energy shortages, and even depression. This leads to productivity losses, a lower sex drive, and, to name a few, anxiety. But still, we are obligated to consume these foods.

What if we could help the mind avoid craving for unhealthy foods? What if we didn't tell the mind when we saw a brownie or chocolate cake that I want to eat a lot of that?

Well, aversion hypnosis is one strategy that is offered by trained hypnotherapists that can help us do just that. It's not always necessary, but it's often one of the most effective solutions for food addiction.

We aren't big fans of aversion therapy for most topics (we'd rather focus our customers on what they want, like a slim healthy body, rather than a negative version of what they don't want, like a cake covered in ants), but when it comes to food and sugar, we find that aversion therapy can be so helpful in tipping the scales for customers that we have to include it here as a possible solution.

Aversion therapy, while creating positive associations with a better option, allows us to create negative associations with something. A hypnotherapist may begin by saying the food is life. Food is natural and derived from nature.

Instead, they might establish a derogatory junk food association (i.e., it's detrimental to us, or even it's poison to our bodies).

Remember The subconscious desires that we feel safe. So when we eat sugary, fatty snacks and light up those reward centers, the subconscious feels we've been given a favor. But it didn't.

Why not for the subconscious, simply? Take the mind away from thinking of processed foods as a reward, or as a comfort blanket – but as a dangerous and unhealthy choice.

Does Food Addictions Hypnosis Work? What Does Research Say

Much of the work on food addiction hypnosis or hypnosis for stopping sugar was conducted around weight loss. And the report is crystal clear. Hypnosis has proved a powerful tool to help people lose weight.

Yes, one study showed that those who used hypnosis on average suffered 20 percent more than those who did not. Additional studies have also found hypnosis to contribute to longer-term outcomes for healthy eating.

Hypnosis has a significant weight loss impact

Researchers investigated how hypnosis could help 60 attendees lost weight in 1986. Hypnosis was used to support ego-strengthening, decision-making, and motivation in the participants. The group that used hypnosis, or 17 pounds to just 0.5 pounds, lost 30 times more on average. (To know more, review our weight loss hypnosis blog!)

Hypnosis The loss of more than 90 percent of others

A meta-analysis of weight loss hypnosis research analyzed 18 studies contrasting cognitive behavioral therapy – i.e., relaxation preparation and controlled imaging – with the same hypnosis-complemented therapies. The results: Hypnosis has helped people lose weight and keep off the weight. Many subjects with hypnosis lost more than 90% of the non-hypnosis community and held it off for two years.

Hypnosis Long Term Weight Loss

One research looked at how hypnosis improved a weight-management treatment plan. One hundred nine participants completed a therapeutic plan in the study, with or without hypnosis. Both groups had lost significant weight after nine weeks. Yet the hypnosis group tended to lose considerable weight at the 8-month and 2-year follow-ups, and it managed to achieve its weight targets.

Start your journey to hypnosis today

Much of the work on food addiction hypnosis or hypnosis for stopping sugar was conducted around weight loss. And the report is crystal clear. Hypnosis has proved a powerful tool to help people lose weight.

Yes, one study showed that those who used hypnosis on average suffered 20 percent more than those who did not. Additional studies have also found hypnosis to contribute to longer-term outcomes for healthy eating.

Hypnosis has a significant weight loss impact

Researchers investigated how hypnosis could help 60 attendees lost weight in 1986. Hypnosis was used to support ego-strengthening, decision-making, and motivation in the participants. The group that used hypnosis, or 17 pounds to just 0.5 pounds, lost 30 times more on average. (To know more, review our weight loss hypnosis blog!)

Hypnosis The loss of more than 90 percent of others

A meta-analysis of weight loss hypnosis research analyzed 18 studies contrasting cognitive behavioral therapy – i.e., relaxation preparation and controlled imaging – with the same hypnosis-complemented therapies. The results: Hypnosis has helped people lose weight and keep off the weight. Many subjects with hypnosis lost more than 90% of the non-hypnosis community and held it off for two years.

Hypnosis Long Term Weight Loss

If you could avoid emotional eating now, what would make your life differently?

Would anyone else notice, or are they just you?

You may wonder how this situation got you. In your mind, you know full well that food is the only thing to do when you 're hungry.

Every other creature on this earth and you know this. It's our way of surviving. You know that eating food when you're not hungry is a formula for discomfort, shame, diminished self-esteem, and weight gain, of course, not just in your brain.

Stop emotional eating? How did it kick-off?

How is it that humans, alone among all the thousands of species of creatures that exist, often seek to fulfill needs that have little to do with bodily hunger for food?

To feel irritated, so instead of coping with what upsets them, head for some pizza in the kitchen. Feeling lonely and mumming on a candy bar instead of finding more social ties. What's the point?

Okay, it is partially because we are so smart. (Ironic, do you not believe?)

We are also the only creatures that use symbols (as far as we know). One thing we can do is stand for another. This is a brilliant skill, and it has allowed us to develop highly sophisticated societies, and to do things that should be very difficult for us on the face of it. But we can and do use the symbols in both negative and positive ways.

This is what happens when we feel an emotional pang, which is like a hunger pang in some ways, so we get somehow reminded of the comfort that comes from eating when we're hungry. Then we make that 'eating comfort' stand-in for whatever it is that would satisfy that emotional need, without really thinking too hard about it. And we're eating.

Tackling the question correctly

You 're going to hear about those horrible feelings of remorse that afflict you after you've indulged in such emotional eating, as though you've done something wrong and you're a bad person somehow. But the culpability is also a consequence of misuse of symbols. It stands in for the real problem, which is that it is not meeting some important needs of yours.

You say this is all very well and very interesting, but how do I get out of it? I did not consciously plan to start eating like this, but I don't seem to be able to stop it, even though I want to!

Hypnosis can help you change old habits

Stop Emotional Eating is a powerful session of audio hypnosis that can help you lose weight and maintain a healthier lifestyle by breaking the grip of this pattern of behavior at the level where it was established-in your unconscious mind.

As you relax and listen to your download over and over again, you will notice several subtle yet significant changes taking place. This you'll find:

Your mind is clearer, and your feelings calmer every time you relax and allow yourself this private time.

You are learning a powerful way of changing the way negative experiences influence you in the present

It begins to feel quite normal to keep the emotional needs and physical needs in your mind very apart-from what you are doing. You begin to find creative ways to deal more effectively with your emotional needs. Eating healthier every day feels natural and normal. You start feeling very good about yourself

hypnotherapy Weight loss

Our specialty is hypnosis for weight loss. When the permanent weight loss procedure of the Gastric Mind Band was introduced over ten years ago, this was to provide a clear alternative to the gastric surgical band.

People who are overweight are increasingly searching for solutions to help them on their weight loss journey. Still, many are reluctant to go for typical gastric band procedures to help build a better relationship with food. Consequently, gastric band hypnosis provides a feasible option, which is healthy and very inexpensive.

Hypnotherapy for weight loss, along with gastric band hypnosis, has become increasingly common and widely available in recent years. People know the many distinct, beneficial effects of hypnotherapy and are therefore much less cynical about these forms of treatments. Let us make it clear at the outset, however, that the Gastric Mind Band Permanent Weight Loss treatment plan, as provided at the Elite Clinic, does not rely solely on hypnosis; it is certainly not what you would normally define as a hypnosis of the gastric bands.

Weight loss hypnosis: Explained

Hypnosis is a state of mind that happens naturally; it is the same state of deep relaxation that you feel when you are about to fall asleep at night. It may also happen while you're dreaming, listening to music or watching a very good movie: when you're concentrating deeply on something important, you can be unaware of what's going on around you, or how much time has gone by.

Gastric band hypnotherapy is the therapeutic use of hypnosis, which is typically carried out in a psychiatric setting to help people make meaningful changes that progress in different areas of their lives. Worded ideas are used by a hypnotherapist to help you solve particular challenges, such as modifying and breaking an unhelpful habit, such as smoking or even chewing your nails. Hypnotherapy can also be used to help you relinquish negative thoughts, build a more optimistic self-image, increase self-esteem, and improve self-assurance.

And how does hypnotherapy, this weight loss, work in the weight loss field? Research results often support the claim that using hypnotherapy/hypnosis in the area of weight loss can be highly effective and help to build a better relationship with your food;, in terms of success, it is comparable with the gastric band. You can read the abstracts Hypnosis efficacy as an adjunct to behavioral weight management, as well as hypnotherapy controlled trial for weight loss in patients with obstructive sleep apnoea.

Overeating hypnosis: Get over your sugar addiction

Do you find yourself reaching during the day for snacks, or at mealtime for extra portions? We 're all doing the same. There comes the point, though, when the habit becomes unhealthy.

Do you want to make a change and end your overeating?

Participants who had hypnosis for overeating reported significant additional weight loss relative to the control group during this study.

Get set to hear more about hypnotic binge feeding! This guide discusses everything you need to decide if hypnotherapy is right for you. Start jumping in and stop your binge eating habit today!

How to confess your food addiction

For overheating, let's think about food addiction before you get a taste of the information around hypnosis. Disordered eating is when you have formed an unhealthy diet- and eating relationship.

Here are some symptoms to watch for that will help you decide whether you have an addiction to food.

Pressure & Never ending the worry

We've all felt pressure — by both the media and our peers — to look at a certain way. Sticking to unrealistic beauty standards, however, can have an impact on your health. You can feel forced to diet, which may lead to anxiety and binge eating.

You may also feel constantly concerned about dieting, eating, and exercising.

If you feel ashamed or guilty about how much you eat, this can add unnecessary pressure to your life.

From dieting to eating disorders

When people feel pressured to look some way by the media, they begin dieting.

But dieting will leave you worrying about food. You can develop disordered eating habits or an eating disorder as a result. This will commit you to a constant diet/binge eating cycle.

The Lasting Process

You'll probably establish an unhealthy eating habit when you become obsessed with food and weight loss. This pattern will leave you constraining yourself, missing meals, eating binge, and then dieting again.

You'll notice constant fluctuations in your weight as you diet yo-yo.

In time, in this endless loop, you might feel like yourself trapped.

The Symptoms

While several different eating disorders occur, the general symptoms include:

- Eating food too quickly
- Continue eating, even if you're full
- Hiding food or feeding in silence
- Feeling forced to eat
- Felt bad after consuming too much
- Eat when you don't feel hungry

Hold your mind on those signs. Hypnotherapy for overeating habits may help if you believe you have a food addiction.

Overeating Hypnosis: How It Works

So, does hypnosis work for overeating?

Yeah! According to this report, patients undergoing overeating hypnotherapy demonstrated greater progress than at least 70 percent of nonhypnotic care clients.

Hypnotherapy will help you conquer an addiction to food. Here are a few ways in which hypnotherapy can help stop us from eating too much.

Mindful Eating

Food addictions cause people to over-eat with little thought. When we fail to think about our actions, it becomes a compulsion.

Hypnosis can teach the mind to stay conscious.

You'll learn how to know your cravings, how full you are already feeling, and how to keep your eating conscious. Mindfulness should make you aware of your actions so that when you feed, you will gain control over how often you consume and how much you feed.

Habit breakers

We develop systematic thinking over time. Binge eating causes us to talk to negative, harmful thoughts about ourselves. We end up eating binge again in response, triggering a relentless cycle of binge eating.

These negative thoughts can cause our cravings, overeating, and stress.

Take a breath during those moments, and remember that everything is okay. Otherwise, the stress becomes anxiety and encourages your binge eating.

To end your food addiction, you must break these negative spirals of thought.

Overeating hypnosis will help you break the habit.

You will take charge of your emotions by using hypnosis. Rather than swimming in the negatives, you'll learn how to make your subconscious a friend (not an enemy).

Treat the Base Condition

Another disorder often triggers food dependency.

You could have depression or an anxiety disorder, for example. Such conditions may cause you to think negatively, which in turn encourages your binge eating.

Hypnosis can empower you and give you the strength of mind you need to fight these conditions. You should take charge and adjust the script, instead of allowing your depression or anxiety to dominate your thoughts.

Treating the underlying disorder will help you break your eating binge habits.

Restore Your Faith

A lack of confidence in oneself can cause us to freeze. Instead of acting or managing our negative feelings, we believe like something is beyond our control.

When we lack self-confidence, our negative thoughts can take over.

Hypnotherapy will help you develop faith in yourself. You can take back control by learning how to believe in yourself. Thus, you can end your unhealthy, eating binge habits.

With overeating hypnotherapy, you will have the confidence to surmount anything.

Techniques for Self-Hypnosis

You should know that you have a few choices available before you continue using hypnotherapy for overeating. For example, one-on-one sessions with a hypnotherapist may be considered. You can also want to listen to the tapes for hypnotherapy.

There is self-hypnosis, as well. Here are some techniques to help get you started:

- ✓ Note your wellbeing and assess how you feel at the start and end of each session
- ✓ Breathe in to tell your mind and body that it is time to relax
- ✓ Count down from 10 which tells your mind that you are in a hypnosis state
- ✓ Talk to yourself using affirmations or constructive advice like "I'm free to over-eat."
- ✓ Imagine taking control of yourself and living a happier, healthier life
- ✓ You can relax with these techniques, and reframe your mind. Application of overeating hypnosis will help you regain control of your eating patterns and daily life.'

- ✓ Binge Eating and Food Addiction hypnotherapy: How it can help

- ✓ Or cravingsHypnosis empowers us to be mindful of our food cravings and teaches the mind how to think about food and how to respond to food.

But just how does that work?

Here's a look at some of the finer binge eating and food addiction hypnosis points, and some of the many ways it can empower us to lead healthier lives.

Mindful Eating:

Nearly all food addictions have a common symptom: Overeating sometimes without thought. It is becoming a habit and something we don't even think about.

They will train the mind to be more conscious of our cravings, how full they feel, and the actual act of eating with hypnosis for mindful feeding. Mindful eating hypnosis allows us to recognize hunger cravings and physical feelings, and to be thoughtful about eating. We are gaining control over food and our cravings.

Breaking Popular Thoughts:

All too often, habitual thinking becomes reactionary and negative. And those thoughts also cause overeating or craving.

You may encounter a stressful situation at work, and instead of taking a breath and saying it's all going to be Fine, you start feeling you 're underqualified, or the stress turns to anxiety.

We can't overcome our food addictions without stopping the spiraling thought patterns.

Hypnosis empowers you to take control of our minds and make a strong friend of our subconscious.

Underlying Conditions to Repair:

Any number of factors can trigger binge eating: Depression, anxiety, lack of self-love, to name a few. Hypnosis can empower us to manage those conditions and move past them.

Restoring Faith:

Lack of self-confidence or love can stop us from acting. If we don't trust ourselves, or if we don't value ourselves, then we can allow our bad habits to continue.

Hypnotherapy is a strong instrument for gaining confidence and learning to love ourselves more. This is important for food addictions. We are much more likely to experience cravings when we love and believe in ourselves and work towards making healthy lifestyle choices.

Chapter 12: THE PSYCHOLOGY OF FOOD CRAVINGS AND EMOTIONAL EATING

Why Do We Have Food Cravings?

One significant factor which may influence appetite control is the thought of food cravings. This urge to devour a specific food seems solid in overweight dieters, and numerous hypotheses has posited why this is so. The nutritional, and homeostatic role of food cravings is described by physiological theories, and explains why cravings might be more present in people who are deprived of food.

The psychoactive abilities of certain foods to trigger cravings are likened to a self-medication behavior and thought to relieve a central serotonin deficits. Psychological theories stress the role of negatives emotions (e.g. anger) as triggers for cravings and learning theories claim that cravings are a positive learnt response to cues (sensory, situational) and giving into a craving results in a pleasurable consequence. What is evident here is that food cravings are a multi-dimensional and complex occurrence, one which possibly involves aspects of all of the proposed theories.

Whatever the reason, it is suggested that food cravings frequently lead to consumption of the craved food and elevated Body Mass Index is associated with food intake and preference for high fat foods. Food craving has been seen to be related to body weight, proposing the significant role of craving in food consumption.

Early identification of elevated body mass indexes (BMI), medical risks, and unhealthy eating and physical activity habits may be essential to the future prevention of obesity. One crucial question is the role food cravings may play in maintaining excessive eating patterns observed in other problems with eating behaviors: binge eating, bulimia, and obesity.

FOOD CRAVINGS AND WEIGHT GAIN: THE MISSING LINK

There is thorough and outstanding evidence regarding the increase in worldwide rates of obesity and the projected outcomes if this is not addressed. Children in particular are noted as being especially at risk of future long term health problems. While dietary restraint, more nutritious eating habits and physical exercise have always been purported to be the answer to the obesity crisis in adults, adolescents and children, long term meta-analysis and follow-up studies indicate that weight loss is not maintained (and indeed the more time that elapses between the end of a diet and the follow-up, the more weight is regained). Unfortunately, several other studies indicate that dieting is actually a consistent predictor of future weight gain.

A recent study conducted by Patricia Goodspeed Grant (2008) involved investigating the psychological, cultural and social contributions to overeating in obese people. She discovered that eating for comfort is rooted in utilizing food to manage experiences of emotional pain.

Her participants revealed that what had been absent from all treatment programs they had attempted was the "opportunity to work on the psychological issues simultaneously with weight reduction". It appears that a missing link in the treatment of overweight and obesity is this concept and issue of addressing the psychological contributors or emotional drivers that are leading people to overeat. Relying on willpower and education is clearly not enough.

Motivation Issues

Humans are only motivated by feelings (i.e. sensations). Basically, there are three (3) types of feelings. These are; pleasant, neutral and unpleasant. The motivation we get from the unpleasant feeling is to move towards a feeling we do not have, but do want. We move away from the unpleasant feeling by replacing it with a different pleasant (or neutral) feeling.

Hunger, is an unpleasant sensation for many people, and it is eased by the pleasant sensation of eating and the taste of food. Most people prefer pleasant sensations compared to unpleasant sensations. But, what we need to know is that pleasant sensations are not always matched with the outcome that they were intended for. Many people eat, not because they need nutrition, but because they feel an unpleasant emotion, like rejection, loneliness, distress, depression, fear, betrayal, worthlessness, defeat, helplessness or hopelessness. This can then create a vicious cycle of more emotional eating to manage the emotional consequences of becoming unhealthy and overweight.

For children, excessive eating and binging are often a consequence of boredom and habit behaviors. Food or drinks are used to relieve the monotony. They can also be used as a coping strategy to deal with problems arising from anxiety, depression, stress and conflicts. Although they may feel comforted after consuming an amount of food, the person has not dealt with the underlying cause of these problems. This sets up a reward cycle of using food to get a better feeling. Consequently, there is no reason why they will not reoccur in the future. This can become a vicious cycle.

If a parent deals with their own emotional issues by eating and or over eating it is highly probable that the child will also do so. This pattern for coping is being modelled. Parents often find it difficult to tolerate their child's disappointment or pain and are motivated to take this away. If food is used regularly as a means of doing this, for example, "Never mind not getting invited let's go get a chocolate sundae," a parent can be setting up a cycle of soothing uncomfortable feelings with the pleasure of food. This ca set up a way of eating to manage feelings or emotion. This is particularly a problem when there is no real discussion of the child's pain or disappointment and instead food is just offered.

Have a think right now: why is it that you want to stop emotionally eating? You might immediately know, or you might have to think for some time.

Your answer/s will give you some insight into how you are motivated.

If you are motivated towards good results, then you might have said some of this to yourself;

• When I quit eating in response to my emotions or feelings, I will be able to purchase clothes 'off the rack' in the shops
• When I quit eating in response to my emotions or feelings, I will be very happy.

If you are motivated away from negative results your answers may reflect:
• When I quit eating in response to my emotions or feelings, I won't be uncomfortable in my clothes any longer
• When I stop eating in response to my emotions I will be able to throw away my 'fat' clothes

You have probably noticed the patterns here. Moving towards pleasurable results or away from a negative one, influences how we think, behave, and feel. You may find out that you have a blend of moving towards certain results and away from others.

This is fine too. More often than not, we are primarily subconsciously motivated in one direction.

Motivation has also been shown to exist either as an internal characteristic or as an external factor in people in general. Inner motivation is connected to neurological circuitry in the left prefrontal lobe. The feelings of achievement, energy for work, excitement in our day all link to the left prefrontal cortex.

It is this area of the brain, which governs motivating behavior. It discourages pessimistic feelings and encourages action. Actually, few people normally possess a significant level of this inner motivation; the individuals who focus on the inner feelings of satisfaction they will attain regardless of any difficulties they face along the way. However others require more than this.

External motivation is any external influence or stimuli to generate positive behavior. These might include monetary rewards such as bonuses, tangible recognition or honor, prizes, or other incentives. The reality is, despite such rewards motivating behavior in the short term, it has been shown that no amount of bonuses or acknowledgment will inspire people to use their fullest potential to keep moving towards their goals. So what does it take?

With exercise, you may have noticed that, regardless the number of fitness coaches you hire, how many motivational exercise tapes you buy, number or classes you attend, in the long run, you lose interest and go back to your old behavior. This is on the ground that those things are forms of external motivation. There is nothing wrong with them, few people thrive on external motivation, and do well at it. However, once in a while, your behavior drops off when you stop getting the drive from an outer source. Let's be honest, if you had a personal fitness coach at your door step every day for the rest of your life, and a personal chef in the kitchen preparing delicious meals forever, then you would be motivated to lose weight, and probably become fitter. Such full time assistance is not a reality for most of us.

Sometimes people discover the inner source of motivation they need to lose weight from an outer source, and this can help them get started.

In 2007, Harvard Medical School's affiliated McLean Psychiatric Hospital did research that showed that Binge Eating Disorder is America's most common eating disorder, far exceeding anorexia and bulimia. The Harvard study clinically defined binging as uncontrolled eating at least twice a week for at least six months. However, experts usually define binging as any episode of uncontrolled eating. A steady diet of overeating and/or binging can lead to all kinds of potential problems. Continual overeating can lead to obesity and a host of other associated diseases such as diabetes, hypertension, elevated cholesterol levels, and certain types of cancers, not to mention the emotional toll it takes. Most binge episodes lead to feelings of guilt, lowered self-esteem and perhaps even depression. So in an effort to enjoy the foods of the upcoming season, and take mindful control over your eating habits, here are tips to handle cravings and avoid overeating.

TIPS TO CONTROL FOOD CRAVINGS AND AVOID OVEREATING

Below are tips to control food cravings and overeating.

1. **Never skip meals or go more than 3-4 hours without eating**.

Uncontrollable cravings and overeating are often the result of extreme hunger. When the body has gone too long without fuel, and blood sugar drops, it's unrealistic to think we can make wise food choices or recognize when we've eaten enough.

2. **Be mindful when eating and learn to use the hunger scale.**

Eating while watching TV, using the computer, talking on the phone or doing any other activity which distract you from your meal, may cause mindless eating and overeating. Eat at your dining table, savoring the smells and tastes of your food. Eat slowly and mindfully, so that you will recognize when you are no longer hungry and feel satisfied. If 1 is completely empty and ravenous, and 10 is feeling like you are in a food coma (stuffed, bloated, exhausted and physically ill), begin eating at 3-4 and stop at 7.

3. **Stop dieting and/or making certain foods completely off limits.**

Most dieters report being obsessed with food thoughts all day, and an increase in cravings for the foods they feel are bad for them. Willpower only goes so far, and most dieters eventually cave into their cravings. Eating mostly healthful, nourishing foods, controlling portions, exercising, and occasionally enjoying a food treat usually accomplishes lasting weight loss.

4. **When craving a food treat, ask yourself, "Am I physically hungry?**

What is it I really want or need?" If you answered "No" to the question of hunger, chances are you are looking to eat for emotional reasons. Loneliness, boredom, anger, frustration, and procrastination are some of the many reasons other than hunger why people eat. If you recognize any of them as your personal triggers, seek help to deal with the underlying causes of your overeating.

5. **Wait out the food craving and distract yourself.**

Most cravings disappear within 10-15 minutes. If you can find something to keep you busy, you might just forget about the craving altogether. Call a friend, read, clean a closet - whatever might absorb you and keep your mind busy.

6. **Try a low-cal or low-fat version of the food you're craving, and use portion-controlled servings.**

Would a small bag of baked potato chips satisfy the urge, or frozen yogurt rather than ice cream? If you feel the need to crunch and munch, would air-popped popcorn satisfy the urge? If it's not a particular food you're after, but a texture or smell, be creative and find a healthier substitute.

7.   **When all else fails, give in to the craving.**

When craving a particular food for hours or even days, giving into it may just be the best strategy. Many an individual have consumed hundreds of calories trying to replace the urge with a "better" choice, only to end up consuming the original craving in the end. Find the absolute best piece of chocolate, or world's leading cheesecake, take a small piece, and savor guilt-free and with pleasure. Enjoying an occasional indulgence cannot destroy a healthy lifestyle.

HOW TO HANDLE FOOD CRAVINGS

Have you had an experience of eating when you are not even hungry? A number of people, including me, often eat when they don't have to. It is unfortunate that feeling hungry is not among the top reasons why people want to eat. Typical reasons could be "seven o'clock is time for dinner in my family", "those cookies look so good" or "those fried chicken smell so yummy". Some researches show that over nine out of ten women have experienced food craving. What is food craving? If you possess a very strong desire to consume a particular food when you are not even hungry, then you have a craving for that food. All of my girlfriends and I belong to the majority of women. Most of my friends have cravings for sweet snacks such as cupcakes, cookies and anything covered with sugar.

Some people don't care for sweet foods, but they often have a craving for salty and spicy snacks. It doesn't matter if they are hungry or not, and they just need to eat salty snack. Once they eat a few, they really feel good and relaxed. It is just so strange. How should people handle cravings? There is no one-size-fits-all solution for everyone. If you have a craving for sweet snacks (which is very common), then you can try low calorie chocolate milk and you might feel satisfied. This have worked for a couple of people, but didn't work for others who claimed that low calorie milk did not fulfill their desire.

When you have a craving for food, allow yourself to have only a limited amount. When you have a craving for some specific foods, you might think eating other things would make the craving go away. This usually doesn't work. You will probably grab the food that you are craving after eating other foods.

Chapter 13: REASONS FOR FOOD CRAVINGS

By far, the two most common types of foods people tend to have cravings for are sugar and high fat foods.

When I say "sugar", I'm talking about all the foods and drinks that convert to sugar in our bloodstream very quickly, not just the obvious things like baked goods, sweets, and candy.

It's also things like refined grains (many would argue that it's "all" grains that are the problem), starchy carbs like bread, pasta, crackers, cereal, bagels, donuts, muffins, pizza, pretzels, granola bars, sports drinks, energy drinks, juice drinks, alcohol, mixes for alcohol, flavored coffee creamers, and so on. The list is rather enormous!

No, the solution is not to substitute with artificial sweeteners, by the way. That's a whole other level of toxicity.

Salty foods are consistently high on the cravings list, too.

So why the cravings?

I consistently find one or more of the following underlying 6 reasons when working with people in various nutritional detoxification and metabolic recovery programs:

1.   Chronic stress

Stress can come from the predictable emotional or mental sources, but it can also come from toxicity in our nutrition or other chemical sources; chronic fatigue; chronic pain; trauma; injury; a lack of proprioception (from movement); environmental issues; medications; illness; autoimmune conditions; etc.

When we are exposed to stress, the brain signals our adrenal glands to release stress hormones, like cortisol and adrenaline. This is a normal response and is perfectly welcome in the short-term fight or flight response. However, many folks are under chronic stress, so the body is burning through major stress hormones on a regular basis.

Two of the main constituents of stress hormones are sugar and fat.

If you're not addressing the source of the stress, the body will continue to do its best to supply you with stress hormones to get you through. In order to do this, it will "demand" that you supply more ingredients for the stress hormones - sugar and fat.

Hence, cravings.

Address the stress, ditch the cravings.

By the way, those adrenals that respond and adapt to stress? When those puppies are over-taxed, that's when we tend to crave salt. If you regularly have salt cravings, check your chronic exposure to stress, your sources of stress, and your response to stress.

2. Bad bugs

If you regularly experience gas and bloating, constipation or diarrhea, headaches, and fatigue along with those sugar cravings, it's an indication that unhealthy bacteria have taken over too much of your gut.

The more advances that are made in science and health research, the more the critical importance of the gut is revealed. It's not "sexy" to talk about the gut, but it's of the utmost importance if you want to live a long, healthy life.

The "gut" comprises vital organs and systems like the stomach, large and small intestines, liver, and gall bladder. Rather significant in the scheme of things, yes?

The human body is truly amazing in its ability to adapt to the toxic abuse we often toss its way, but there are consequences to this abuse, whether we see or feel the effects of it now or not. This proliferation and over-growth of unhealthy bacteria in the gut is actually quite common, considering how vulnerable gut bacteria are to environmental assaults.

The healthy bacteria of our gut need to be there. They are a vital component of our health on many levels. They keep the overall "flora" of the gut in check.

Our lifestyle choices influence our gut flora on a daily basis. In particular, our gut is very sensitive to: antibiotics, chlorinated and fluoridated water, pesticides and other agricultural toxins, antibacterial soaps and cleaners, poor diet, and much more.

It may be a challenge to have direct control of your community's water supply or what's being sprayed on crops in your county, but you certainly have control over many components of your diet.

These unhealthy, pathogenic bacteria, and yeast, and fungi love a steady supply of sugar. In fact, it nourishes them. This proliferation of bacteria and yeast has been described by some doctors as actually causing more harm than elevated blood sugar and insulin resistance, which are very serious problems.

Yeast is a normal and natural part of our bodies when it's in a state of balance.

When yeast grows out of control, it's referred to as Candida or Candidiasis. Candidiasis is notorious for causing sugar cravings. Why? Because it feeds on sugar!

Remember that list of foods that convert to sugar very quickly in our bodies? Sigh. Those are the enemy, especially if you have yeast/Candida issues.

Typically, by temporarily removing sugar from the diet for a few weeks to a few months, most people can restore a healthy balance of yeast. (Often, they also need to incorporate #3 below to have lasting success.)

Again, until the source of the problem is addressed, it's hard to battle those cravings with just your determination and will.

Stop feeding the Candida, ditch the cravings.

3. Gut permeability issues

This component is huge. It's also very closely related to the first two reasons. Funny how the body works like that!

Here's the really simple, nutshell version of what's going on:

The lining of the intestines forms a life-saving barrier for us. When this lining is damaged, we end up with intestinal permeability, or "leaky gut". Now, food particles that are far too large are passing through the barrier right into our bloodstream. This is definitely not good.

The immune system does its thing, goes on the attack and responds to this invader. If the gut is not repaired properly, then the heightened immune response continues. In some cases, an autoimmune response is created - where the immune system attacks the body's own tissue.

Again, until the cause is addressed, the problem will continue.

When the gut lining has been damaged (due to the typical North American lifestyle - poor diet, toxicity, chronic stress, drugs/medication, environmental factors like mold, pesticides, heavy metals like mercury in dental fillings and vaccines, etc.), the body doesn't receive the nutrients it needs.

The vast majority of nutrient assimilation takes place in the small intestines. If it's damaged, the body won't get what it needs.

Hence, the potential for cravings.

Heal the gut, ditch the cravings.

When you diligently work to repair gut issues in the proper way, along with removing the source(s) of toxicity and eating a "proper diet" that continues to nourish and heal (that includes traditionally fermented foods known to help heal the gut lining), not only should cravings subside, but overall health and vitality will dramatically improve.

4. Hormonal Imbalance

This is too large of a topic to fully dive into here, but I'll give you a taste.

Hormones are little chemical messengers - they're like little cars traveling throughout our bodies, carrying various messages for every function in the body. They need a place to park. The hormone receptors (garages for the cars, if you will) line the cell membranes of every single cell in our body.

In order for healthy function to unfold, the cars need to park in the garages so that the messages can be transferred to the cell.

When cells become "congested" due to many of the same factors that interfere with a healthy gut (listed in #2 and #3), the garages are blocked or altered so that the cars can't deliver the message. In addition to throwing physiological function off in a major way, this resulting "hormonal imbalance" can cause food cravings.

We can try to artificially add more hormones (cars) to the mix, but that's generally not the problem. The problem is the garage doors (cell membrane and hormone receptors). This is true for all hormones - whether we're talking reproductive hormones, or thyroid hormones, or anything in between.

Fix the cell membrane, detoxify the cell, and ditch the cravings.

5. Excitotoxins

Again, the simplified version: excitotoxins are food additives that are considered "neurotoxins", meaning they are toxic to our brain and nervous system.

Some of the common excitotoxins you may recognize are MSG (monosodium glutamate), aspartame, hydrolyzed proteins, and autolyzed yeast, as well as ingredients listed as "natural flavors" and "spices".

These additives "enhance" the taste of foods, making us crave these new, "exciting" flavors, rather than the old, boring ones that real foods provide. They change the expectations of our taste buds!

Eat real food without all the additives, ditch the cravings.

6. Drugs

I have come to learn in our practice experience that, when things just are just plain wacky with a patient, when their symptoms are all over the place, breaking all the rules, oftentimes it's due to their medications. The pharmaceuticals that people take now are a new, disturbing breed, causing a dizzying array of side effects.

One of these side effects can be food cravings. (Honestly, it's probably the least of your concerns with the dangerous side effects that these drugs could be causing!)

Talk to your prescribing doctor(s) about an exit strategy for all drugs that are not currently keeping you alive! In the overwhelming majority of cases, you should not "have to" take a drug for life. That would mean that the drug is not fixing anything, right?

Make the changes necessary to sustain your own life, as well as your health.

Dump the drugs, ditch the cravings. Live long and prosper!

Chapter 14: HARNESSING POSITIVE AFFIRMATION AND MEDITATION FOR WEIGHT LOSS.

Positive Affirmation for weight loss

I know that feeling. You're putting too much energy into it, and you've made considerable attempts to lose extra weight, but it doesn't work out as you expect. What if I tell you that simple values may be detrimental to your endeavors. Those positive affirmations will change everything.

You know what, when you feel that you've stuck a spot in your weight, you've put it into the mirror and it's very difficult to see what you're doing, you feel i in literally uncomfortable in your clothing. The feeling of being discouraged, frustrated, and depressed because you have put too much effort and followed certain guidelines to say things are happening but and it makes you think you should eat more and more of course many have developed eating disorder from their high school days and pursued it through to adulthood.

But the good news is this, these poor eating habits have been changed by other people who have access to quality knowledge and key points as we lay open to you in this book.

It's interesting to know that those who think they've constantly stopped eating have no change or shift in their thoughts and emotional experience about food yet. This then trips too often over the body. It is more like going from being weighty and progressing to being overweight in panic. There are also negative perceptions and thoughts towards the body and an unhealthy food relationship. By healing them you can change your body image. Then, you love your body, and you develop a healthy food relationship.

These ten systems of beliefs are keys to the underlying unyielding forces that have been in the subconscious mind. Should we go through these ten affirmations, please. Together we will see what exactly represented the underlying factor that helped to hinder your weight loss. It may be as simple as flipping your odd faith to affirmative, by harnessing certain positive beliefs, in which you set yourself up for success. It is high time you converted all the demoralizing, destructive, and restricting beliefs into positive ones, as you identify them and expose them, as you see things happening and improving.

The affirmations that have been highlighted are those I have seen work people into reality of their results.

1. Affirmation such as "I am lean and healthy"

The first thing you need is your confidence and how you see your body. You 're at the point between, "I want to be healthy and lean." Go ahead and declare it as a fact, not just as a wish. Let your body system start digesting those words in. Just as you have pronounced and declared, start living in the excitement and joy of spoken truth, your living in this understanding and conviction is your real energy.

The fact that what you do doesn't look like what you say doesn't mean you 're self-deceptive. You are just trying to establish within you the truth you want, and you believe it will materialize. You are now not living in your hideous state of mind but in the modern. Live the Truth you profess about yourself in the moment. This is what builds the factor of your self-identity. When you believe in this truth, your body, one way or the other starts living from the inside out in that sense. May I tell you the body is capable of conforming to this truth.

2. I place high esteem to myself over food.

It's best to place focus on yourself rather than food. Do a good job of testing how much you treat the body and using the food as compensation. We also think less about what our needs are, but what kind of food, what style of food, what measure of food, how delicious it is, how satisfying it will be, all these and more are what we think and focus our minds on at the expense of maintaining our body.

This has literally been ties spanning from our childhood. When we buy "special food" from our parents as a reward for doing well in school or for getting good results. Over time, these ideas have formed the foundation of our belief system. At adulthood too, we feel, when we get promoted from the office or when your wife goes to bed or something good happens. We seem to eat excessively and most times use food as a means to celebrate these achievements even to the detriment of our wellbeing. Going this way with unhealthy relationship with food is so detrimental.

3. Affirmation such as "I love my body"

Therefore, growing beyond the relevance of food to body relevance is required of you. You eat well to shape your body and you're not building your body for the food. So, it is body food and not food body. Simply declare to yourself that "I love my body and fat just left ." Therefore, when you look into the mirror and you put it down sluggishly and hurriedly, you make some words and even statements to yourself. The question then is, can you tell your intimate pal that you very much appreciate what you just said to yourself when you look at the mirror?

Your body systems are all hears, listening quietly to your confessions on them. It's high time I told you to love your body

This junk is circulated through our experiences; what if I chose to love and see my body in a way that I don't like? Doesn't it mean that I'm just flattering myself or does it mean that I just have to love my body even though I know it won't improve or make any difference, I don't care what's going on with the body, I just have to love it.

This is not the idea, the idea is where there is growth, where there is love, there is development, there are greater tendencies for change. When you show some love to your body, it's inspired to change. But if you believe otherwise by being self-humiliated and shameful, then you assume that you overeat.

4. Affirmation such as "I have my perfect weight"

Go to the mirror again and guess what? Say to yourself, this is how I am and I will enjoy it like this now "I will certainly harness the potency of love to strengthen, maintain and evoke the necessary change in my body.

Claim to yourself saying, I am my ideal weight. How long and far I'm going to go in saying what I'm not, No, that's not you just have to build and fashion for yourself. You know what ? If you don't believe, you can't see it.

5. Affirmation such as "I am super cool in my clothes".

I feel good and comfortable in my clothes. It sounds uncomfortable and unrealistic, isn't it? The problem that arises in your mind is; how can I pretend to feel comfortable and nice in a dress that is out of size when the clothes on me are not fitting.

The real thing is, you've just got to choose the size you 're aiming for to the weight you're now. In dressing up your truth to the physical. You only have to build the impression of fitness on clothes, otherwise any cloth does not appear to fit you.

6. Affirmation such as " I wave away foods that are unhealthy for me"

One of the wrong style to eating or poor relationship with food is by checking, how many foods you say yes to that are practically unhealthy.

What if you said no easily? Be deliberate about it and do not regret saying it, for it will end in good news. Don't waste money on food which is destructive to you, invest in affirmations instead.

7. Affirmative like "I am glued to body enhancing foods and materials"

At this, we are wrestling psychologically with two things. The old self and the new self, old belief and new belief, old and new feelings, old and new life, old relationships and new relationships with food. Both of these are steps that need to be left for the other. First of all, you don't have to feel a sense of denial about what the sense of denial is when you're on the road to making life good for you, or maybe better.

8. Affirmation such as "I am satisfied with the necessary amount of food"

This is so amazing, because it regulates and exposes you to how much you consume and how much you would eat. Many people just stop eating hen when the food is not finished not when they are satisfied; other people only have to eat to the fullest before taking their hands off the food. It should not work like this, because it is an unhealthy eating style. That's it; say "I 'm done," "I'm satisfied, "I had enough".

WEIGHT LOSS AFFIRMATIONS

To find your ideal weight, you need to heal all aspects of yourself. You need to heal with regular exercise, a mindful presence, natural food, and the spiritual nourishment of self-compassion.

For all the wrong reasons, many of us eat until we feel full, seeking satisfaction through food by consuming while we are emotional or bored. Eating for any reason other than nourishment need has created a well-worn path of bad habits.

Here's my proposal. Suppose you have an abundant supply of self-fulfilment through a creative outlet, a life full of spiritual nourishment, purpose, and self-love. In that case, you are already "full," and satisfaction through food becomes less significant. In this case, we are fulfilled by an inner sense of calm and security, so we simply eat for nourishment and fuel.

Genuine change begins in mind and begins with a thought. Reprogramming the mind by eliminating negative thinking that developed the bad health habits in the first place is important, and it is a realistic way to apply Eckhart Tolle's words, "Get the inside right and the outside falls in place."

Below are 90 affirmations that can help with mindful weight loss. Utilize one of them, some of them, or all of them!

1. I have a plan to lose weight, and I intend to stick to that plan.
2. I'm determined to reach my goal weight.
3. I'm completely committed to losing the extra weight.
4. My weight is not necessarily what defines me.
5. I take care of my body, always.
6. I am motivated to lose weight and get healthy.
7. I'm fully committed to losing weight.
8. I'll always respect and care for my body.
9. I believe that I can lose weight.
10. I'm going to think positively and naturally lose weight.
11. Just as my reasons to hold on to my extra weight slip away, so does the weight.
12. I am shedding the extra pounds today, thus shredding my self-doubt.
13. Nothing stands between me and my target weight today, and I mean nothing.
14. I lose weight every day, and the people around me are taking notice.
15. I love and cherish myself t my present weight, even as I march pound by pound to my target weight.
16. My weight loss lies inside of me. My diet is just a tool to get me right to my goal.
17. I choose to stay on the path.

18. I eat foods that complement my new weight.
19. Each day I get stronger and slimmer.
20. I'm ready and determined to lose weight.
21. I am supported by people around me in the weight loss process.
22. I can accomplish anything I put my mind to.
23. Attaining my weight loss goal is getting easier every day.
24. Losing weight helps me feel comfortable and more confident in my skin.
25. I 'm giving myself the healthy, strong body I deserve.
26. I am losing weight daily.
27. I am becoming stronger and fitter daily through exercise.
28. I 'm constantly cultivating more healthy eating habits.
29. I'm happily exercising every morning when I wake up, so I can reach the weight loss I want.
30. By changing my eating habits, I commit myself to my weight loss program.
31. In my great effort to lose weight, I am pleased with every part I do.
32. It's so exciting to discover my unique weight loss food and exercise system.
33. I'm a kind person. I deserve love. It 's safe for me to lose weight.
34. For every single day, I get closer and closer to my ideal weight.
35. I can do this; my body is losing weight right now.
36. I am the strongest version of myself, and I work hard to make myself even better. I'm going to lose weight because I want to, and I've got the power to do so.
37. I can achieve my weight loss goals, and I won't let anything stay in my way.
38. I enjoy being physically fit because I lose weight enough to be at my ideal weight.
39. I 'm losing all the extra weight in my body and mind and feeling light.
40. My weight loss journey is joyful and perfect.
41. I have the power to turn my life around.
42. I'm achieving my goals on weight loss. I do energy-generating and fat-burning workouts regularly, I actively chose to eat healthily, and I live in a state of NOW mindfulness.

43. I will overcome. My mind is taking charge of my body. Injury does not slow me down. I'll find a to achieve my goals for weight loss.
44. I reach my weight loss goals because I appreciate the food's pros and cons, and I choose to consume nutritious food and reap the positive results it brings and my weight loss results.
45. My mind and bodywork together in harmony to help me achieve success in terms of balance, serenity and weight loss.
46. My body is a temple. I'm cautious of only putting in good things that will keep the system running smoothly and help me meet my weight loss goals.
47. I am the master of my body, and mind-I am disciplined and will achieve my weight loss goals.
48. I love my body, and I appreciate everything that it does for me. I now feed it with foods that nourish it and let it lose excess weight effortlessly.
49. I only eat healthy food when I'm hungry, and I easily lose weight. I love my body.
50. The weight that I no longer need leaves my body right away.
51. I lose weight every single day.
52. Weight loss feels great.
53. I've taken control of my weight loss.
54. I'm fast approaching my weight loss goal.
55. I think weight loss, so I lose weight.
56. My behavior and actions support my ideal weight.
57. I find it easy to lose weight now.
58. I am now losing weight regularly and healthily.
59. I lose weight and move more quickly towards my ideal weight now.
60. I make choices that help my weight-loss journey.
61. I always picture myself at my ideal weight.
62. I've got whatever it takes to lose weight and reach my ideal body weight.
63. All the weight I lose, I lose forever.
64. I truly love my body, which helps me in my weight loss journey.
65. I am intensely motivated to reach my weight loss goal.
66. I 'm committed to a healthy lifestyle that is not only good for weight loss but also greater self-esteem and self-confidence.
67. I dwell on all the positive long-term effects that my weight loss will bring me.

68. I set myself realistic but challenging goals which inspire me to lose weight and feel great.
69. My drive and focus never waver on my weight loss journey.
70. My heart and soul are so passionate and driven to my goals of weight loss academic achievement.
71. Not only is my health improving, but my entire life is also changing. And it feels amazing!
72. I have confidence in myself to make the right choices that will create great weight loss.
73. I give thanks for having a body that's able to work out and lose weight effectively.
74. My core values are around my weight loss journey, helping me make better choices.
75. Everyone is different, and to my weight loss, I hold no expectations, only that it is and will continue to happen.
76. The entire universe conspires to help me lose weight and lose fat.
77. I love setting new goals for myself that keep me motivated and inspired to keep my weight loss going.
78. All my emotions and feelings around my weight loss are predicated.
79. I commit to slow and healthy weight-loss, for this is the secret to sustainable weight loss in the long term.
80. I have all the mental and physical strength required for a long-lasting and successful weight loss.
81. I dwell on the positive weight loss aspects.
82. I find a reason why I want to lose weight. Strong enough to get me through those tough times.
83. I allow my intuition to guide me on better health and weight loss process.
84. I see weight loss as a marathon rather than a sprint. So naturally, I make choices that benefit my health in the long term.
85. Through this journey of weight loss, I awaken the giant within me.
86. I see fitness and weight loss as a journey, not a destination.
87. I know my mind is strong, so I listen and watch things that make my mind stronger—helping my journey down weight loss.
88. Through my positive commitment to weight loss, I love how my entire life has changed.

89. Failure is only feedback. I learn from my weight loss failures and use them to make me better.
90. Naturally, my old bad habits fall away and are replaced by healthy habits which make my weight loss easy.

Chapter 15: HYPNOTHERAPY PLAN FOR 12 WEEKS

A 12-week hypnotherapy program was the most effective product we found for weight reduction.

The program takes on some commitment as each of the hypnosis recordings was split right into twelve sessions, among which it is necessary to listen to them daily.

• Week one

You'll be provided with the foundations for your brand-new weight management regime in the very first week of the hypnotic course. In addition to setting your weight-loss target, you are also skillfully guided to eliminate a lot of your self-imposed limiting ideas around your ability to produce and maintain a healthy, balanced, non-fat, and fit body.

• Week two

In the second component of the course, you learn exactly how to determine the very own all-natural signals from your body. If you're hungry, your body will let you know! Your body lets you know when you are full! You'll learn how to distinguish between an urge and the intake.

However, when you use hypnotherapy to conquer this irrational belief in what to eat, you can ensure that your everyday food intake is greatly reduced.

• Week three

To change your mental patterns and practices, Neuro-Linguistic Programming (NLP) is used. NLP is a set of approaches designed to produce rapid behavioral improvements that are highly successful and clinically verified.

If used along with hypnosis, NLP provides quick, long-term promotion of behavioral change.

• Week four

You are making use of hypnotic sessions to direct your memory back to your over-eating primary source, then removing the causes that leave you without emotional consumption.

• Week five

You are mentally trained to drink plenty of water within week five. Water is an incredible aid in weight loss since it fills you up. Intake of water reduces the pangs of cravings. It also has terrific health and wellness benefits and gets rid of the body's contaminants.

• Week six

You are trained in these sessions to integrate gentle, natural exercise right into your daily routine to increase your metabolic rate and slim down more quickly.

Hypnotherapy can be an important help in any form of weight-loss plan and has been revealed very quickly to produce some amazing results. Weight loss by hypnosis is not a "magic disk." Coupled with a regular weight loss routine or diet routine and exercise plan, it is convincing. Water is a great aid in weight loss because it will fill you up.

• Week seven

You're conditioned to start eating more healthily at this point in the training course.

- Week eight

This is designed to help you raise your metabolic price by gaining direct access to your subconscious mind and changing the plan for your body that it holds. Even though, as we said earlier, other hypnotic CDs may try this method, it works in this course because you are already conditioned to take more workout!

The hypnotic ideas used this week will surely help you get even more out of your exercise regimen and thus burn fat faster!

- Week nine

As you move closer throughout the hypnotic course of weight loss, you'll surely use the Swish method to make sure the brand-new practices you've discovered become irreversible.

- Week ten

Now it's time to take advantage of your subconscious mind's ability to help you burn even more fat. By using hypnotic pointers effectively, you can command your subconscious mind to consume more of the fat that is kept in your body. The training course will transform your consuming habits and the level of exercise even more!

- Week eleven

This week deals with the critical self-image problem! By ensuring that you have a positive self-image and a healthy and balanced respect for your body, you will ensure that you remain healthy and balanced, and do not abuse your brand-new weight-loss ability!

- Week twelve

Your program's Week 12 coatings. Currently, you should see major emerge from the work you've done before. Recommendations are provided which enhance your new practices and keep you motivated to maintain a healthy, balanced fit body.

The use of hypnotherapy as a quick fix option is not going to work for your weight problems! Using it as an instrument to help you shed weight could be the difference between success and failure. If you want to shed weight completely and truthfully and develop a safe and balanced body, then hypnosis is most certainly a way to make the necessary adjustments simple, long-term, and fast.

As this is a 12-week hypnotic training course covering all weight-loss aspects, it is not the most affordable choice available. Even though you can get more affordable one-session alternatives, they will at best give you average results.

The program is a behavioral-change system designed to help you achieve your perfect weight and make the adjustment irreversible. Because it changes your behavior and attitude towards food and exercise, at the subconscious level, once you finish the course, it just feels all-natural to preserve your brand-new healthy and balanced overview and consumer and workout practices!

CONCLUSION

What is the relationship between Hypnosis and weight-loss? Hypnosis is something that we like to find as a kind of fun, but have you ever thought of weight-loss Hypnosis? It is trying to use Hypnosis to cope with a situation as extreme as weight issues, so maybe it's not as crazy as it seems. Weight-loss Hypnosis is an enticing concept-it gives people a fairly easy way out of their weight issue by preventing their appetite for food at the source.

One weight-loss dilemma by Hypnosis is the same issue that affects other approaches to weight-reduction.

There are plenty scams out there, and the people behind them do not hesitate to try to take your money for a product that does nothing at all. Hypnosis does have the same problem. You may be able to trust some statements regarding weight-loss therapy for Hypnosis; however, there are just as many who have loads of lies.

If weight-loss treatment hypnosis declares it can help you lose some insane number of pounds in a few weeks or similar exaggerations, it is pretty safe to bet it's a scam. If you find claims that say that Hypnosis can alter the way the mind works to avoid eating, they are likely to be deceiving.

As you sleep or wake up from sleep, your mind goes through the various stages of brainwave operation. Bata's where you're now if you don't dream, that's it. The waves are high. There is Alpha just under that knowledge. The waves are slower and awake but in a modified state of consciousness. Have you ever driven your car, and you're just thinking about your questioning where you were at the exit? Yeah, when driving, you've got your mind attached to the Alpha zone. When under Hypnosis, this is the same thing the brain does. Keep in mind when driving the car that you kept in control, that you hit nothing, that's the same with Hypnosis. Theta comes under the Alphah; you don't sleep but go to sleep. And you're unconscious, known as the Delta. When you get up, you are going in reverse through those brainwave states.

Now that we understand the workings of our minds let's start talking about Hypnosis. Hypnosis is the workaround within the conscious mind of the vital dimension and the establishment of embracing discerning thoughts. Notice that the definition does not say something about relaxing or giving up control? Hypnosis is more of a natural condition.

Always read a book and sort of slip off in your mind anywhere else? If answered yes to any of these concerns, then you were previously hypnotized. Some always say it's like daydreaming, but I prefer to disagree.

Daydreaming is typically when your mind thinks of something, thinks of being on a boat, or some other particular circumstance or scene. As I drive my car and fall into that "pace," I know my mind is completely blank, I don't think anything. By looking at a dot on the wall, you will go into Hypnosis.

The fact is, Hypnosis will help you lose weight. Hypnosis is more science than magic; what it is when a person finds himself in a state of intense, relaxed focus where he becomes more suggestive.

A hypnosis session won't turn you into some sort of device that's immune to yearnings and not programmed to overindulge. However, what this can do is make a person more likely to follow a proper dietary strategy. The effects are psychological entirely. Hypnosis can not "persuade" your body to promote weight loss; it can only implant the idea into your brain that you do not need to eat the second piece of cake.

Individuals seeking hypnotic weight loss therapies should be very cautious about group hypnosis sessions. For order to function, Hypnosis has to be precisely adapted to the person who gets it. Group sessions will not work, as the therapist can not connect on his own with any single person. You should also be warned against cassettes or videos of Hypnosis since they share this same issue.

Weight-reduction Hypnosis is an enticing idea. If you can train your mind to minimize your yearnings and increase your self-discipline, then you will be well on your way to weight loss.

Be vigilant and research all the alternatives before you buy an item or see a hypnotherapist, or else you will end up with nothing at all, is the crucial thing to keep in mind.

Have you ever experienced Hypnosis before? NO, then let me tell you a little bit about Hypnosis and what you might expect to feel, just to relax your mind and help you get the most out of this incredibly powerful kind of help.

As I said, "hypnosis" comes from a Greek term, "Hypnos," meaning sleep (you could not sleep).

After reading this book, I hope I've helped you explore some of the initial questions you posed at the beginning and also provided thought-provoking answers!

What I love about the idea of mindful eating is how it can allow us to re-center and refocus on our part of the day; otherwise, we would not give a second thought about it.

Like a lot of people, I am guilty of quickly grabbing a sandwich and munching on the go without really understanding my nutritional needs, both physical and mental.

Bringing a little awareness of the picture can help us find deeper fulfillment and gratitude for our eating habits, which can lead to a stronger sense of health as well.

Are you tired of suffering emotional eating and overeating?

Are you looking for a plan to heal your body and mind?

Do you want effortlessly lead a healthy life and achieve your dream body?

You've already noticed that eating a nutritious breakfast will save you from cravings later in the day and will potentially help you shed the extra weight that you've been carrying around for some time now goals you set .The hypnosis of weight loss is, therefore, real and is now helping individuals from all walks of life achieve their weight loss goals and give them control of their lives by giving them a safe and easy way to achieve their desired level of health.

in this book you will learn :

- TIPS TO BUILDING A PLAN FOR LASTING SUCCESS
- 10 TRICKS FOR SEEING WEIGHT LOSS FAST RESULTS
- BUILDING A GOOD RELATIONSHIP WITH FOOD
- ADDITIONAL TIPS FOR MAINTAINING AN HEALTHY RELATIONSHIP WITH FOOD
- EXPLORING THE MIND BODY CONNECTION WITH HYPNOSIS
- UNDERSTANDING THE POWER OF BELIEF IN WEIGHT
- SIMPLE WAYS TO QUICKLY BOOST YOUR SELF-ESTEEM
- 30 KNOWN WAYS THAT WEIGHT LOSS WILL CHANGE YOUR LIFE
- 18 WAYS TO MINIMIZE HUNGER AND APPETITE BASED ON SCIENCE
- LOVE YOURSELF WHEN LOSING WEIGHT
- 5 THINGS TO REMEMBER AFTER WEIGHT LOSS ABOUT BODY IMAGE
- UNDERSTANDING HYPNOTHERAPY GASTRIC BAND
- WHAT IS EMOTIONAL NUTRITION?
- HOW GASTRIC BAND HYPNOSIS PERFORMS
- 5 STUFF YOU DIDN'T HEAR ABOUT HYPNOTHERAPY GASTRIC BAND
- BASIC AND ADVANCED VIRTUAL GASTRIC BAND WEIGHT LOSS PROGRAMS
HOW DOES MEDITATION RELATE TO FOOD AND WEIGHT   LOSS

- WEIGHT LOSS MEDITATION BENEFITS
- THE MINDFULNESS APP
- THE PLANET'S 20 MOST WEIGHT LOSS FRIENDLY FOODS

- THE GUIDE FOR HEALTHY EATING
- HOW TO MAINTAIN HEALTHY EATING
- WHAT IS AN ADDICTION TO FOOD?
- 8 COMMON FOOD ADDICTION SYMPTOMS HOW TO USE MINDFULNESS FOR WEIGHT LOSS
- THE TOP 10 REASONS TO USE HYPNOTHERAPY WEIGHT LOSS
- ERRORS IN WEIGHT LOSS YOU NEED TO STOP MAKING
- THE BENEFITS OF CONSCIENTIOUS EATING
- HOW TO PRACTICE FOOD MINDFULNESS
- STOPPING FOOD ADDICTION

The program is a behavioral-change system designed to help you achieve your perfect weight and make the adjustment irreversible. Because it changes your behavior and attitude towards food and exercise, at the subconscious level, once you finish the course, it just feels all-natural to preserve your brand-new healthy and balanced overview and consumer and workout practices! So what are you waiting for? Scroll up and buy now!!